Primary Sclerosing Cholangitis

INTERNATIONAL FALK WORKSHOP

Primary Sclerosing Cholangitis

EDITED BY

M. P. Manns
Department of Gastroenterology
and Hepatology
Zentrum Innere Medizin
Medizinische Hochschule Hannover
Carl-Neuberg-Str. 1
D-30625 Hannover
Germany

R. W. Chapman
Department of Gastroenterology
John Radcliffe Hospital
Headington
Oxford
UK

A. Stiehl
Medizinische Klinik
Klinikum der Universität
Bergheimer Str. 58
D-69115 Heidelberg
Germany

R. H. Wiesner
Gastroenterology Unit
Mayo Clinic and Foundation
200 First Street SW
Rochester, MN 55905-0001
USA

Proceedings of the International Falk Workshop (Part II of the Liver Week in Freiburg 1997) held in Freiburg, Germany, October 3, 1997

KLUWER ACADEMIC PUBLISHERS
DORDRECHT / BOSTON / LONDON

Distributors

Sold and distributed in North, Central and South America by Kluwer Academic Publishers, PO Box 358, Accord Station, Hingham, MA 02018-0358, USA

In all other countries, sold and distributed by Kluwer Academic Publishers, Distribution Centre, PO Box 322, 3300 AH Dordrecht, The Netherlands

A C.I.P. Catalogue record for this book is available from the Library of Congress.

ISBN 0-7923-8745-7

Printed on acid-free paper

Published by Kluwer Academic Publishers PV, PO Box 17, 3300 AA Dordrecht, The Netherlands.

Printed in Great Britain by MPG Books Ltd, Bodmin, Cornwall

Contents

SECTION III: NON-SURGICAL TREATMENT

List of Principal Authors

U. Broomé
Department of Gastroenterology and Hepatology
Huddinge University Hospital
S-14186 Huddinge
Sweden

R.W. Chapman
Department of Gastroenterology
John Radcliffe Hospital
Headington
Oxford
OX3 9DU
UK

P.T. Donaldson
Institute of Liver Studies
King's College Hospital
Denmark Hill
London
SE5 9RS
UK

U. Hopf
Medizinische Klinik und Poliklinik Charité
Campus Virchow-Klinikum
Humboldt-Universität zu Berlin
Augustenburger Platz 1
D-13353 Berlin
Germany

K. Huibregtse
Academisch Ziekenhuis
University of Amsterdam
Academisch Medisch Centrum
Meibergdreef 9
NL-1105 AZ Amsterdam Zuidoost
The Netherlands

M.M. Kaplan
New England Medical Center Hospitals
Gastroenterology Division, Box 233
750 Washington Street
Boston
MA 02111-1533
USA

J. Ludwig
Center for Basic Research in Digestive Diseases
Guggenheim 17
Mayo Clinic
200 First St. SW
Rochester
MN 55905
USA

M.P. Manns
Department of Gastroenterology and Hepatology
Zentrum Innere Medizin
Medizinische Hochschule Hannover
Carl-Neuberg-Str. 1
D-30625 Hannover
Germany

J.M. Neuberger
The Liver Unit
The Queen Elizabeth Hospital
Queen Elizabeth Medical Centre
Edgbaston
Birmingham
B15 2TH
UK

E. Schrumpf
Medical Department A
Section of Gastroenterology and Hepatology
Rikshospitalet
Pilestredet 32
N-0027 Oslo
Norway

A. Stiehl
Medizinische Klinik
Klinikum der Universität
Bergheimer Str. 58
D-69115 Heidelberg
Germany

J.M. Vierling
Center for Liver Diseases and Transplantation
Cedars-Sinai Medical Center
8635 West Third Street, Suite 590W
Los Angeles
CA 90048
USA

S. Wagner
Abteilung für Gastroenterologie und Hepatologie
Zentrum für Innere Medizin
Medizinische Hochschule Hannover
Carl-Neuberg-Str. 1
D-30623 Hannover
Germany

R. Wiesner
Gastroenterology Unit
Mayo Clinic and Foundation
200 First Street SW
Rochester, MN 55905-0001
USA

R. Williams
Institute of Hepatology
University College London Medical School and Hospitals
69–75 Chenies Mews
London
WC1E 6HX
UK

Preface

Primary sclerosing cholangitis is a disease of unknown cause. It is regarded as one of the autoimmune liver diseases, although this still needs to be proven. Furthermore, primary sclerosing cholangitis is a systemic disorder rather than a pure liver disease. Among the many diseases associated with primary sclerosing cholangitis, inflammatory bowel disease is the most prominent one. Up to 80% of patients with primary sclerosing cholangitis suffer from inflammatory bowel disease, in particular ulcerative colitis. One of the severe complications of primary sclerosing cholangitis is bile duct cancer. Advances in primary sclerosing cholangitis include our knowledge of the natural history, immunopathogenesis, genetics, medical treatment such as ursodesoxycholic acid, endoscopic treatment by dilation of prominent bile duct stenoses, and surgical treatment, in particular liver transplantation. In the past, this fascinating disease has been underdiagnosed. An International Falk Workshop, totally devoted to the different aspects of primary sclerosing cholangitis, was held in Freiburg, Germany, on October 3, 1997. Internationally renowned experts gathered in Freiburg to discuss current knowledge of epidemiology, pathogenesis, diagnosis and treatment of this intriguing disease that still leaves us with so many questions. Roger Chapman, Adolf Stiehl, Russell Wiesner and I are very grateful to all members of the faculty and the discussants attending the International Falk Workshop. We are particularly grateful to all the authors of the various chapters of the proceedings, which give us a comprehensive and up-to-date overview of primary sclerosing cholangitis.

M.P. Manns, *Hannover*
R.W. Chapman, *Oxford*
A. Stiehl, *Heidelberg*
R.H. Wiesner, *Rochester*

Section I
Diagnosis, aetiology and pathogenesis

1
Primary sclerosing cholangitis: diagnosis and differential diagnosis

K. M. BOBERG and E. SCHRUMPF

INTRODUCTION

Primary sclerosing cholangitis (PSC) is a generalized disease of the intrahepatic and/or extrahepatic bile ducts, characterized by inflammation and fibrosis with development of bile duct strictures. It follows a chronic but variable course with eventual progression to liver cirrhosis. Delbet[1] was the first to report a documented case of sclerosing cholangitis in 1924. In the early descriptions of PSC, the diagnosis was based on findings at laparotomy consisting of pathological bile ducts with thickening of the bile duct wall due to a diffuse sclerosing and stenotic process[2–5]. Intraoperative cholangiograms revealed irregularities, narrowing and strictures of the extrahepatic as well as the intrahepatic bile ducts[5]. The introduction of endoscopic retrograde cholangiography (ERC) made visualization of the bile duct tree more accessible, and ERC is now the major diagnostic tool in PSC[6,7].

PSC must be distinguished from secondary sclerosing cholangitis due to other disorders. In addition to the findings of generalized sclerosis and stenosis of the bile ducts, the traditional criteria for the diagnosis of PSC include: (1) absence of previous biliary surgery; (2) absence of gallstones; and (3) exclusion of carcinoma of the bile ducts[3,4]. The observation that PSC patients are predisposed to development of biliary tract calculi[8] as well as cholangiocarcinoma[9] should, however, be taken into consideration. In combination with the typical cholangiographic findings, the diagnosis of PSC is based on clinical, biochemical, and histological data (Table 1).

DIAGNOSIS OF PSC

Patient history and clinical features

The typical PSC patient is a young male with inflammatory bowel disease (IBD) who presents with a cholestatic biochemical pattern. There is a male predominance in this disease with a male to female ratio of approximately

Table 1 The diagnosis of PSC is based on:

Patient history and clinical findings
Biochemical and serological findings
Liver histology
Cholangiography

2:1[10–14]. The majority of the patients are diagnosed in their thirties[10–15], but there is a wide range from childhood[16] to old age[14]. Typically, there is a delay from the first biochemical sign or symptom of liver disease until the diagnosis of PSC is verified[13,14]. In a group of 305 Swedish patients, the median age at diagnosis was 39 years (range 5–80) with a median delay of 52 months (range 0–451) from the first biochemical or clinical sign compatible with PSC[14].

The clinical history up to the time of diagnosis of PSC varies considerably. Some patients are asymptomatic and are referred for investigation due to increased serum alkaline phosphatase (ALP) levels, most often in the presence of concomitant IBD[10–20]. Other patients present with symptoms of liver disease, ranging from mild to severe, with signs of liver cirrhosis and portal hypertension[10–20]. The proportion of asymptomatic patients at diagnosis varies between different studies from 10–25%[10–12,20] up to 44%[13,14]. This variation may partly be explained by differences in patient selection, but may also be attributed to differences in the definition of symptoms[14]. Symptomatic patients most commonly experience jaundice, pruritus and upper right abdominal pain[10–15,21]. More unspecific symptoms, like weight loss, fever, and fatigue, are also reported. Some patients may have had episodes of acute cholangitis[10]. Signs of portal hypertension with ascites and variceal haemorrhage may occur, but are less frequent at the time of diagnosis. Physical examination at diagnosis was abnormal in 50% of the patients investigated by Wiesner and LaRusso[11], with jaundice, hepatomegaly and splenomegaly as the most prevalent findings.

The symptoms in PSC may be intermittent, and, notably, some patients who are initially symptomatic may be asymptomatic at a later investigation. In the study by Schrumpf *et al.*[13], 21 among 43 symptomatic patients were asymptomatic at follow-up at a median of 6.2 years after the diagnosis. Some of the asymptomatic patients may remain so for several years[13,20–22]. Some authors describe a more benign disease course with a prolonged survival in the asymptomatic patients compared with the symptomatic group[14,20]. In other studies, there is no significant difference in the prognosis between asymptomatic and symptomatic patients[12,13,23,24], underlining the progressive nature of PSC, also in the asymptomatic group.

Biochemical and serological findings

Biochemical tests in patients with PSC usually show a cholestatic profile. Serum ALP activity is elevated in the majority of the patients, often to a level at least three times the upper normal limit[10–15]. An increased ALP activity in a patient with IBD is frequently the first evidence for PSC, but an elevated ALP level is not a prerequisite for the diagnosis. Up to 8.5% of the patients in large studies

Table 2 PSC must be distinguished from secondary sclerosing cholangitis due to:

Previous biliary surgery
Cholelithiasis
Tumours of the bile ducts
Immunodeficiency disorders
Viral infections
Ischaemia

have had normal ALP levels at diagnosis[14]. In a group of 12 patients with normal ALP activity at diagnosis of PSC, advanced cholangiographic and histological changes were present in 4 cases[25]. The ALP activity may also fluctuate and return to normal during periods of the disease course[25]. As a consequence, a normal ALP value should not preclude further steps to diagnose PSC if suspected on a clinical basis, particularly in a patient with IBD.

Most PSC patients have a moderate elevation of the transaminase levels to about 2–3 times upper normal values. Serum bilirubin concentration is within normal limits in up to 60% of patients at diagnosis[14,15,20,21]. The mean bilirubin concentration in studies of large patient groups varies from 16 to 68 μmol/L[12–15]. As the disease progresses, bilirubin levels may gradually increase, but there may also be fluctuations caused by bile duct sludge and stones or intermittent episodes of bacterial cholangitis. The synthesis function of the liver is intact in the majority of patients at the time of diagnosis, with normal levels of albumin and coagulation factors[10–15].

PSC patients may have increased levels of circulating immunoglobulins and positive titres of autoantibodies. In a study of 114 PSC patients, the IgG concentration was elevated above upper limits of normal in 61%[26]. In a large proportion (44%), the IgG level was up to 1.5 times the upper normal limit, but, in a few patients (5%), the IgG concentration was higher than twice the upper normal limit. Increased IgM levels have been observed in 20–45% of patients[10,17]. Antinuclear antibodies (ANA) and smooth muscle antibodies (SMA) may be detected but less frequently and in lower titres than in autoimmune hepatitis (AIH)[10,17,26,27]. Antimitochondrial antibodies (AMA) are rare in PSC[2,11,26]. PSC in childhood is also associated with elevated levels of immunoglobulins and positive titres of ANA and SMA[28,29].

Perinuclear antineutrophil cytoplasmic antibodies (pANCA) are detected in the serum of 26–85% of PSC patients[30–32]. Since pANCA is also found in sera from patients with other chronic liver disorders, like primary biliary cirrhosis (PBC) and AIH[31–33], this test is not specific for PSC and its role as a diagnostic marker in this disease has not been established.

Liver histology in PSC

The most prominent histological changes in liver biopsies from PSC patients are located in the portal tracts featuring inflammation, periductal fibrosis, ductal obliteration, bile duct proliferation or loss of bile ducts in later stages[34–36]. Parenchymal changes with piecemeal necrosis, focal necrosis, focal inflammation, Kupffer cell hyperplasia and perilobular fibrosis may also be present[10,21,34].

Four histological stages have been defined[34], and it is believed that the disease process in PSC progresses through these stages with eventual development of cirrhosis.

Stage 1 (portal stage) is characterized by portal oedema, mild portal hepatitis and ductal proliferation. There may be a mild non-destructive cholangitis with infiltration of lymphocytes in the bile ducts. Parenchymal changes tend to be mild or absent[34].

In stage 2 (periportal stage or stage of portal enlargement), the lesion extends to involve periportal fibrosis and inflammation, sometimes with piecemeal necrosis of periportal hepatocytes. The portal tracts are often enlarged. There may be ductular proliferation, periductal fibrosis and fibrous–obliterative cholangitis. Periductular fibrosis is considered highly suggestive of PSC[34]. Development of portal-to-portal fibrous septa characterizes the stage 3 lesion (septal stage). Bile ducts degenerate and disappear. Stage 4 is the cirrhotic endstage, showing the regenerative nodules, often accompanied by ductular proliferation and oedema in the periphery[34].

None of the histological findings in PSC are pathognomonic, and a definite diagnosis must be established by ERC.

Cholangiography

The diagnosis of PSC relies on typical cholangiographic findings by ERC or percutaneous transhepatic cholangiography, including bile duct mural irregularities and diffusely distributed multifocal strictures[6,7] (Figure 1). Usually, both the intrahepatic and extrahepatic bile ducts are involved but isolated intrahepatic changes have been described in up to >20% of cases[20,37]. Since abnormalities of the intrahepatic bile ducts may also be seen in other chronic liver disease, one must be cautious when diagnosing PSC in the presence of intrahepatic changes only. Multiple strictures of the extrahepatic biliary tree together with normal intrahepatic ducts are detected in some patients[10]. The bile duct strictures in PSC are typically short and annular with intervening normal or dilated segments, resulting in a pattern of 'beading'. Sometimes the dilatations may have a diverticular appearance[7]. Long confluent strictures may be seen with more advanced disease. Development of cirrhosis results in approximation and tortuosity or a stretched and displaced appearance of the intrahepatic bile ducts[7]. The gallbladder and cystic duct are involved in about 15% of cases[35].

Abnormalities of the pancreatic ducts, resembling those of chronic pancreatitis, are visualized in a variable number of the PSC patients[7,38,39].

DIFFERENTIAL DIAGNOSIS IN PSC

PSC must be distinguished from other hepatobiliary disorders which may present with cholestasis like primary biliary cirrhosis (PBC) and drug-induced reactions, but also including cases of autoimmune hepatitis (AIH), alcoholic hepatitis, and viral hepatitis with a cholestatic biochemical profile[40]. Cholangiographic features resembling those of PSC have been reported in various immunodeficiency states,

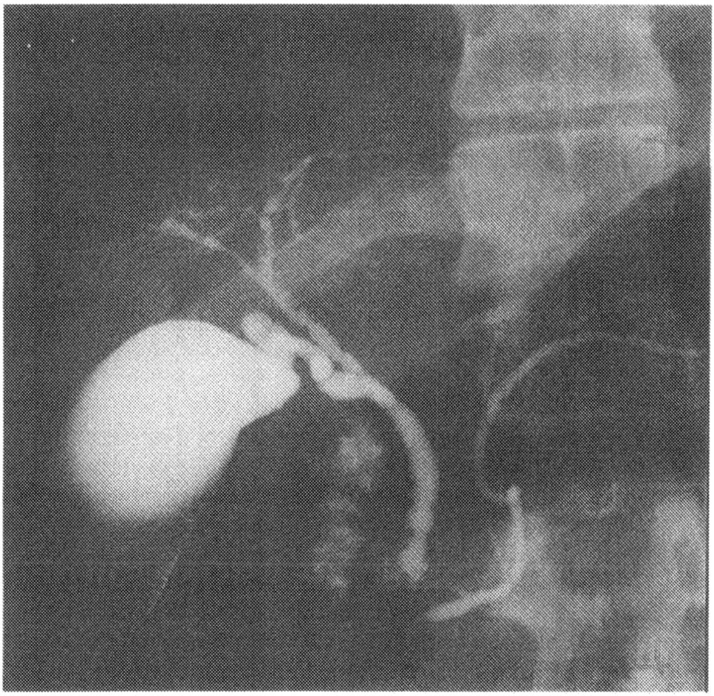

Figure 1 Typical cholangiographic findings in PSC

like the acquired immunodeficiency syndrome and in association with certain viral infections, like cytomegalovirus infection[41]. Ischaemia secondary to hepatic artery injury or injection of toxic substances may lead to fibrosis and strictures of the bile ducts[42,43]. Bile duct obstruction caused by choledocholithiasis, tumours, or surgical trauma must be excluded as a cause of secondary sclerosing cholangitis (Table 2). In most cases, patient history, serological and virological tests, and liver histology will contribute to the correct diagnosis.

Some important differential diagnostic problems encountered in the clinical situation will be presented in the following (Table 3).

Hepatobiliary lesions in ulcerative colitis

PSC is associated with inflammatory bowel disease in up to about 90% of cases[44,45]. The majority of patients have ulcerative colitis (UC) but there is also an association with Crohn's colitis[44]. Evidence of hepatobiliary disorders has been reported in 3–15% of patients with UC[18,19,46–49]. PSC is the single most frequent hepatobiliary lesion in UC and is diagnosed in 2.1–4% of the cases. The prevalence of PSC in UC may be as high as 7.5% in selected patient groups[49].

Liver biopsies from patients with UC reveal a spectrum of histological

Table 3 Difficult differential diagnoses when PSC is suspected

Cirrhosis with or without intrahepatic PSC
Cirrhosis with or without small-duct PSC
Autoimmune hepatitis or PSC (large- or small-duct PSC)
Autoimmune hepatitis with or without PSC (large- or small-duct PSC)
Autoimmune cholangitis or PSC (large- or small-duct PSC)

abnormalities, including fatty changes, portal inflammation and fibrosis, pericholangitis, chronic active hepatitis, cirrhosis, and cholangiocarcinoma[18,19,46,50,51]. The cholangiographic findings in UC may also vary[52]. Some of the hepatobiliary lesions in UC may thus be difficult to distinguish from PSC. Pericholangitis may be described with or without concomitant characteristic cholangiographic features of PSC. Ludwig[53] has suggested that the term 'pericholangitis' should be replaced by 'small-duct PSC', affecting only microscopically identifiable interlobular and septal bile ducts, as opposed to large-duct PSC with cholangiographic changes of the extrahepatic and large intrahepatic bile ducts. They further proposed that the clinical diagnosis of small-duct PSC should be based on: (1) typical liver biopsy findings; (2) biochemical abnormalities similar to those in (large-duct) PSC; and (3) the presence of one or two accompanying conditions, namely IBD (in particular UC) or large-duct PSC, or both. Accordingly, a patient presenting with UC, a cholestatic biochemical profile, liver biopsy findings compatible with PSC, but with a normal cholangiogram, should be diagnosed as having a small-duct PSC[53]. In a study of 18 patients with ulcerative colitis and similar clinical, biochemical, and histological findings to those of PSC, 5 patients had a normal ERC of the both the extrahepatic and the intrahepatic bile ducts[54]. In the remaining 13 patients, intrahepatic abnormalities were noted, but these were different from classical intrahepatic changes in PSC. They comprised long biliary stenoses, approximation of the intrahepatic ducts, and decreased arborization[54]. It was suggested that all these 18 patients should be classified as having small-duct PSC[54]. Small-duct PSC and classical PSC probably represent different aspects of the same disease spectrum, but better diagnostic criteria are needed.

Autoimmune hepatitis

PSC patients may have biochemical, histological, and clinical features resembling those of AIH[10,11,17,34]. The concurrence of PSC and AIH in the same patient has been suggested in some cases[55–58]. Elevated levels of circulating immunoglobulins and non-organ-specific autoantibodies and the presence of interface hepatitis in liver biopsies in some patients may be difficult to differentiate from the findings in AIH. Treatment with corticosteroids may, at least temporarily, induce biochemical and clinical improvement in selected cases[26]. A markedly increased serum transaminase activity and less prominent ALP elevation, together with a sustained response to immunosuppressive therapy, would favour a diagnosis of AIH. When 114 PSC patients were assessed according to a scoring system for the diagnosis of AIH[59], 2% of the patients could be classified as 'definite' AIH and 33% as 'probable' AIH[26]. This finding emphasizes the importance of performing ERC in the differential diagnosis between PSC and AIH. Among the 114 PSC patients, five carried a diagnosis of AIH for several years before PSC was diagnosed by ERC. In particular, in patients with IBD, one should be reluctant to diagnose AIH until ERC has excluded PSC[49]. Whether a patient may suffer from both PSC and AIH simultaneously and should be given both diagnoses, has not been widely discussed and agreed upon. Until specific histological findings and/or serological tests for the two conditions have been established, this question will be difficult to resolve.

Primary biliary cirrhosis and autoimmune cholangitis

Patients with PBC also present with cholestasis and may clinically be difficult to differentiate from PSC[60]. The diagnosis is usually established by the presence of AMA and typical histological features with a chronic, destructive cholangitis of the small intrahepatic bile ducts[61]. The histological findings may sometimes be difficult to distinguish from those of PSC, in particular in the late disease stages[62]. AMA-positivity supports the diagnosis of PBC in such cases, since this finding is far less frequent in PSC[26,54]. About 5–10% of patients with biochemical and histological features of PBC lack AMA and may contribute to the differential diagnostic problems in chronic liver disease[61–63]. The majority of the AMA-negative patients are positive for ANA (often in high titres)[63,64]. They are also more frequently SMA positive but have significantly lower IgM levels than AMA-positive patients. The term 'autoimmune cholangitis' or 'autoimmune cholangiopathy' has been proposed to denote this patient category[63–65].

Detection of antibodies to the enzyme carbonic anhydrase which is abundant in the bile duct epithelium, has been suggested as a test to distinguish between various immune-mediated liver diseases[66]. In the study by Gordon *et al.*[66], antibodies to carbonic anhydrase were frequent in the sera of patients classified as having autoimmune hepatitis, but uncommon or not present in patients with AMA-positive PBC, PSC and AIH. These results could not be confirmed by others[67]. In summary, the autoantibody status may be unreliable as a diagnostic tool in the differentiation between the various autoimmune liver disorders. ERC should be carried out to confirm the diagnosis of PSC when this remains a possibility. In patients with normal cholangiograms, small-duct PSC remains a possible diagnosis, and the distinction between small-duct PSC and autoimmune cholangitis may be difficult or even impossible.

Cirrhosis

The development of cirrhosis in PSC leads to cholangiographic changes in the intrahepatic bile ducts as seen in cirrhosis of any aetiology[34]. The differentiation of patients with intrahepatic PSC and cirrhosis from other cirrhotic patients may therefore be impossible on the basis of cholangiography. Further improvement of the cholangiographic technique may partly solve this problem, but most likely, in the future, differential diagnosis will depend upon the establishment of other diagnostic tests in tissue or blood samples.

Cholangiocarcinoma

PSC patients carry an increased risk of developing cholangiocarcinoma[9–14,68,69]. The reported frequencies of cholangiocarcinomas associated with PSC range from 6% up to about 30%[9–14,68,69]. Most often, cholangiocarcinoma develops in a patient with a known diagnosis of PSC, but, in some cases, the two conditions present at the same time. Among 30 patients reported from the Mayo Clinic[9], the diagnosis of PSC preceded that of cholangiocarcinoma by a mean of 52 months in 21 patients, whereas simultaneous diagnoses of PSC and cholangiocarcinoma were made in 9 patients. It has been argued that a diagnosis of cholangiocarcinoma excludes that of PSC and that the bile duct changes in these cases are secondary to the tumour infiltration[9]. There is, however, evidence that cholangiocarcinoma in these cases develops in the setting of PSC in patients with ulcerative colitis[70,71].

The clinical differentiation between PSC alone and PSC complicated by cholangiocarcinoma may be extremely difficult and represents a diagnostic challenge. Often cholangiocarcinoma is not detected until laparotomy in connection with liver transplantation or at autopsy. Certain cholangiographic features may raise the suspicion of cholangiocarcinoma[52,71,72], and brush cytology of such areas may increase the diagnostic sensitivity[49,73]. Histological findings of bile duct epithelial dysplasia in liver biopsy specimens have been associated with development of cholangiocarcinoma[74] but its significance has to be further investigated. Ultrasonography and computerized tomographic (CT) scanning should be performed, but cholangiocarcinomas may not be detected by these techniques. Rapid onset of persistent jaundice, pruritus and weight loss, associated with a marked rise in bilirubin and ALP, may indicate development of malignancy[9,75] but are unspecific findings which may also be seen in PSC patients without cholangiocarcinoma. In several reports, neither clinical findings, biochemical tests, nor prognostic indices have identified patients with cholangiocarcinoma[13,68,76].

High levels of the tumour-associated antigen, CA 19-9, in serum are present in up to 80–90% of PSC patients with concurrent cholangiocarcinomas, and CA 19-9 has been suggested as a diagnostic marker of malignancy, alone or in combination with carcinoembryonic antigen[77,78]. CA 19-9 is not specific since it may also be increased in patients with benign disease[79], and its role in screening for cholangiocarcinoma in PSC is at present unclear[77].

CONCLUSION

If PSC is suspected and ERC is performed, the diagnosis of PSC is easily established in most cases. In a small proportion of the patients (Table 3), the differentiation between PSC and closely related disorders may be very difficult and, in some cases, impossible. Specific diagnostic tests for PSC, either in bioptical specimens or in blood samples, are urgently needed.

References

1. Delbet MP. Rétrécissement du cholédoque. Cholécysto-duodenostomie. Bull Mem Soc Nat Chir. 1924;50:11446.
2. Schwartz SI, Dale WA. Primary sclerosing cholangitis. Review and report of six cases. AMA Arch Surg. 1958;77:439–51.
3. Holubitsky IB, McKenzie AD. Primary sclerosing cholangitis of the extrahepatic bile ducts. Can J Surg. 1964;7:277–83.
4. Warren KW, Athanasiades S, Monge JI. Primary sclerosing cholangitis. A study of forty-two cases. Am J Surg. 1966;111:23–38.
5. Thorpe MEC, Scheuer PJ, Sherlock S. Primary sclerosing cholangitis, the biliary tree, and ulcerative colitis. Gut. 1967;8:435–48.
6. Ayoola EA, Vennes JA, Silvis SE, Rohrmann CA, Ansel HJ. Endoscopic retrograde intrahepatic cholangiography in liver diseases. Gastrointest Endosc. 1976;22:156–9.
7. MacCarty RL, LaRusso NF, Wiesner RH, Ludwig J. Primary sclerosing cholangitis: findings on cholangiography and pancreatography. Radiology. 1983;149:39–44.
8. Kaw M, Silverman WB, Raninovitz M, Schade RR. Biliary tract calculi in primary sclerosing cholangitis. Am J Gastroenterol. 1995;90:72–5.
9. Rosen C, Nagorney DM, Wiesner RH, Coffey RJ, LaRusso NF. Cholangiocarcinoma complicating primary sclerosing cholangitis. Ann Surg. 1991;213:21–5.
10. Chapman RWG, Arborgh BÅM, Rhodes JM *et al.* Primary sclerosing cholangitis: a review of its clinical features, cholangiography, and hepatic histology. Gut. 1980;21:870–7.
11. Wiesner RH, LaRusso NF. Clinicopathological features of the syndrome of primary sclerosing cholangitis. Gastroenterology. 1980;79:200–6.
12. Farrant JM, Hayllar KM, Wilkinson ML *et al.* Natural history and prognostic variables in primary sclerosing cholangitis. Gastroenterology. 1991;100:1710–17.
13. Schrumpf E, Abdelnoor M, Fausa O, Elgjo K, Jenssen E, Kolmannskog F. Risk factors in primary sclerosing cholangitis. J Hepatol. 1994;21:1061–6.
14. Broomé U, Olsson R, Lööf L *et al.* Natural history and prognostic factors in 305 Swedish patients with primary sclerosing cholangitis. Gut. 1996;38:610–15.
15. Okolicsanyi L, Fabris L, Viaggi S *et al.* Primary sclerosing cholangitis: clinical presentation, natural history and prognostic variables: an Italian multicenter study. Eur J Gastroenterol Hepatol. 1996;8:685–91.
16. Wilschanski M, Chait P, Wade JA *et al.* Primary sclerosing cholangitis in 32 children: clinical, laboratory, and radiographic features, with survival analysis. Hepatology. 1995;22:1415–22.
17. Schrumpf E, Fausa O, Kolmannskog F, Elgjo K, Ritland S, Gjone E. Sclerosing cholangitis in ulcerative colitis. A follow-up study. Scand J Gastroenterol. 1982;17:33–9.
18. Schrumpf E, Elgjo K, Fausa O, Gjone E, Kolmannskog F, Ritland S. Sclerosing cholangitis in ulcerative colitis. Scand J Gastroenterol. 1980;15:689–97.
19. Shepherd HA, Selby WS, Chapman RWG *et al.* Ulcerative colitis and persistent liver dysfunction. Q J Med. 1983;208:503–13.
20. Helzberg JH, Petersen JM, Boyer JL. Improved survival with primary sclerosing cholangitis. A review of clinicopathologic features and comparison of symptomatic and asymptomatic patients. Gastroenterology. 1987;92:1869–75.
21. Aadland E, Schrumpf E, Fausa O *et al.* Primary sclerosing cholangitis: a long term follow-up study. Scand J Gastroenterol. 1987;22:655–64.
22. Chapman RWG, Burroughs AK, Bass MN, Sherlock S. Long-standing asymptomatic primary sclerosing cholangitis: report of three cases. Dig Dis Sci. 1981;26:778–82.
23. Lebovics E, Palmer M, Woo J, Schaffner F. Outcome of primary sclerosing cholangitis. Analysis of long-term observation of 38 patients. Arch Intern Med. 1987;147:729–31.
24. Wiesner RH, Grambsch PM, Dickson ER *et al.* Primary sclerosing cholangitis: natural history, prognostic factors and survival analysis. Hepatology. 1989;10:430–6.
25. Balasubramaniam K, Wiesner RH, LaRusso NF. Primary sclerosing cholangitis with normal serum alkaline phosphatase activity. Gastroenterology. 1988;95:1395–8.
26. Boberg KM, Fausa O, Haaland T *et al.* Features of autoimmune hepatitis in primary sclerosing cholangitis: an evaluation of 114 primary sclerosing cholangitis patients according to a scoring system for the diagnosis of autoimmune hepatitis. Hepatology. 1996;23:1369–76.
27. Zauli D, Schrumpf E, Crespi C, Cassani F, Fausa O, Aadland E. An autoantibody profile in

primary sclerosing cholangitis. J Hepatol. 1987;5:14–18.
28. El-Shabrawi M, Wilkinson ML, Portmann B *et al.* Primary sclerosing cholangitis in childhood. Gastroenterology. 1987;92:1226–35.
29. Mieli-Vergani G, Lobo-Yeo A, McFarlane BM, McFarlane IG, Mowat AP, Vergani D. Different immune mechanisms leading to autoimmunity in primary sclerosing cholangitis and autoimmune chronic active hepatitis of childhood. Hepatology. 1989;9:198–203.
30. Duerr RH, Targan SR, Landers CJ *et al.* Neutrophil cytoplasmic antibodies: a link between primary sclerosing cholangitis and ulcerative colitis. Gastroenterology. 1991;100:1385–91.
31. Klein R, Eisenburg J, Weber P, Seibold F, Berg PA. Significance and specificity of antibodies to neutrophils detected by western blotting for the serological diagnosis of primary sclerosing cholangitis. Hepatology. 1991;14:1147–52.
32. Seibold F, Weber P, Klein R, Berg PA, Wiedmann KH. Clinical significance of antibodies against neutrophils in patients with inflammatory bowel disease and primary sclerosing cholangitis. Gut. 1992;33:657–62.
33. Bansi DS, Bauducci M, Bergqvist A *et al.* Detection of antineutrophil cytoplasmic antibodies in primary sclerosing cholangitis: a comparison of the alkaline phosphatase and immunofluorescent techniques. Eur J Gastroenterol Hepatol. 1997;9:575–80.
34. Ludwig J, LaRusso NF, Wiesner RH. Primary sclerosing cholangitis. In: Peters RL, Craig JR, eds. Liver Pathology. New York: Churchill Livingstone; 1986:193–213.
35. Lee Y-M, Kaplan MM. Primary sclerosing cholangitis. N Engl J Med. 1995;332:924–33.
36. Barbatis C, Grases P, Shepherd HA *et al.* Histological features of sclerosing cholangitis in patients with chronic ulcerative colitis. J Clin Pathol. 1985;38:778–83.
37. Bhatal PS, Powell LW. Primary intrahepatic obliterating cholangitis: a possible variant of 'sclerosing cholangitis'. Gut. 1969;10:886–93.
38. Epstein O, Chapman RWG, Lake-Bakaar G, Foo AV, Rosalki SB, Sherlock S. The pancreas in primary biliary cirrhosis and primary sclerosing cholangitis. Gastroenterology. 1982;83:1177–82.
39. Børkje B, Vetvik K, Ødegaard S, Schrumpf E, Larssen TB, Kolmannskog F. Chronic pancreatitis in patients with sclerosing cholangitis and ulcerative colitis. Scand J Gastroenterol. 1985;20: 539–42.
40. Harnois DM, Lindor KD. Primary sclerosing cholangitis: evolving concepts in diagnosis and treatment. Dig Dis. 1997;15:23–41.
41. Sherlock S. Pathogenesis of sclerosing cholangitis: the role of nonimmune factors. Semin Liver Dis. 1991;11:5–10.
42. Terblanche J, Allison HF, Northover JMA. An ischemic basis for biliary strictures. Surgery. 1983;94:52–7.
43. Kemeny M, Battifora H, Blayney DW *et al.* Sclerosing cholangitis after continuous hepatic artery infusion of FUDR. Ann Surg. 1985;202:176–81.
44. Fausa O, Schrumpf E, Elgjo K. Relationship of inflammatory bowel disease and primary sclerosing cholangitis. Semin Liver Dis. 1991;11:31–9.
45. Quigley EMM, Beaver SJ, Wiesner RH, LaRusso NF. Familial occurrence of liver disease and inflammatory bowel disease in primary sclerosing cholangitis. Gastroenterology. 1987;92:A149.
46. Dew MJ, Thompson H, Allan RN. The spectrum of hepatic dysfunction in inflammatory bowel disease. Q J Med. 1979;189:113–35.
47. Olsson R, Danielsson Å, Järnerot G *et al.* Prevalence of primary sclerosing cholangitis in patients with ulcerative colitis. Gastroenterology. 1991;100:1319–23.
48. Broomé U, Glaumann H, Hellers G, Nilsson B, Sörstad J, Hultcrantz R. Liver disease in ulcerative colitis: an epidemiological and follow up study in the county of Stockholm. Gut. 1994;35: 84–9.
49. Schrumpf E, Fausa O, Egjo K, Kolmannskog F. Hepatobiliary complications of inflammatory bowel disease. Semin Liver Dis. 1988;8:201–9.
50. Eade MN. Liver disease in ulcerative colitis. I. Analysis of operative liver biopsy in 138 consecutive patients having colectomy. Ann Intern Med. 1970;72:475–87.
51. Wee A, Ludwig J. Pericholangitis in chronic ulcerative colitis: primary sclerosing cholangitis of the small bile ducts? Ann Intern Med. 1985;102:581–7.
52. Kolmannskog F, Aakhus T, Fausa O *et al.* Cholangiographic findings in ulcerative colitis. Acta Radiol (Diagn). 1981;22:151–7.
53. Ludwig J. Small-duct primary sclerosing cholangitis. Semin Liver Dis. 1991;11:11–17.
54. Boberg KM, Schrumpf E, Fausa O *et al.* Hepatobiliary disease in ulcerative colitis. An analysis of 18 patients with hepatobiliary lesions classified as small-duct primary sclerosing cholangitis. Scand J Gastroenterol. 1994;29:744–52.

55. Minuk GY, Sutherland LR, Pappas SC, Kelly JK, Martin SE. Autoimmune chronic active hepatitis (lupoid hepatitis) and primary sclerosing cholangitis in two young adult females. Can J Gastroenterol. 1988;2:22–7.
56. Rabinovitz M, Demetris AJ, Bou-Abboud CH, Van Thiel DH. Simultaneous occurrence of primary sclerosing cholangitis and autoimmune chronic active hepatitis in a patient with ulcerative colitis. Dig Dis Sci. 1992;37:1606–11.
57. Lawrence SP, Sherman KE, Lawson JM, Goodman ZD. A 39 year old man with chronic hepatitis. Semin Liver Dis. 1994;14:97–105.
58. McNair ANB, Molony MM, Portmann BC, McFarlane IG, Williams R. Natural course of autoimmune hepatitis (AIH) overlapping with primary sclerosing cholangitis (PSC) in six patients. Hepatology. 1996;24:232A.
59. Johnson PJ, McFarlane IG. Meeting report: International Autoimmune Hepatitis Group. Hepatology. 1993;18:998–1005.
60. Wiesner RH, LaRusso NF, Ludwig J, Dickson ER. Comparison of the clinicopathologic features of primary sclerosing cholangitis and primary biliary cirrhosis. Gastroenterology. 1985;88:108–14.
61. Sherlock S, Scheuer PJ. The presentation and diagnosis of 100 patients with primary biliary cirrhosis. N Engl J Med. 1973;289:674–8.
62. Batts KP, Ludwig J. Histopathology of autoimmune chronic active hepatitis, primary biliary cirrhosis, and primary sclerosing cholangitis. In: Krawitt EL, Wiesner RH, eds. Autoimmune Liver Diseases. New York: Raven Press, Ltd; 1991:75–92.
63. Lacerda MA, Ludwig J, Dickson ER, Jorgensen RA, Lindor KD. Antimitochondrial antibody-negative primary biliary cirrhosis. Am J Gastroenterol. 1995;90:247–9.
64. Michieletti P, Wanless IR, Katz A *et al.* Antimitochondrial antibody negative primary biliary cirrhosis: a distinct syndrome of autoimmune cholangitis. Gut. 1994;35:260–5.
65. Ben-Ari Z, Dhillon AP, Sherlock S. Autoimmune cholangiopathy: part of the spectrum of autoimmune chronic active hepatitis. Hepatology. 1993;18:10–15.
66. Gordon SC, Quattrociocchi-Longe TM, Khan BA *et al.* Antibodies to carbonic anhydrase in patients with immune cholangiopathies. Gastroenterology. 1995;108:1802–9.
67. Heathcote J. Autoimmune cholangitis. Gut. 1997;40:440–2.
68. Abu-Elmagd KM, Selby R, Iwatsuki S *et al.* Cholangiocarcinoma and sclerosing cholangitis: clinical characteristics and effect on survival after liver transplantation. Transplant Proc. 1993; 25:1124–5.
69. Farges O, Malassagne B, Sebagh M, Bismuth H. Primary sclerosing cholangitis: liver transplantation or biliary surgery. Surgery. 1995;117:146–55.
70. Wee A. Ludwig J, Coffey RJ Jr, LaRusso NF, Wiesner RH. Hepatobiliary carcinoma associated with primary sclerosing cholangitis and chronic ulcerative colitis. Hum Pathol. 1985;16:719–26.
71. Mir-Madjlessi SH, Farmer RG, Sivak MV. Bile duct carcinoma in patients with ulcerative colitis. Relationship to sclerosing cholangitis: report of six cases and review of the literature. Dig Dis Sci. 1987;32:145–54.
72. MacCarty RL, LaRusso NF, May GR *et al.* Cholangiocarcinoma complicating primary sclerosing cholangitis: cholangiographic appearances. Radiology. 1985;156:43–6.
73. Rabinowitz M, Zajko AB, Hassanein T *et al.* Diagnostic value of brush cytology in the diagnosis of bile duct carcinoma: a study in 65 patients with bile duct strictures. Hepatology. 1990;12; 747–52.
74. Martins EBG, Fleming KA, Garrido M, Hine KR, Chapman RWG. Superficial thrombophlebitis, dysplasia, and cholangiocarcinoma in primary sclerosing cholangitis. Gastroenterology. 1994; 107:537–42.
75. Miros M, Kerlin P, Walker N, Harper J, Lynch S, Strong R. Predicting cholangiocarcinoma in patients with primary sclerosing cholangitis before transplantation. Gut. 1991;32:1369–73.
76. Broomé U, Eriksson LS. Assessment for liver transplantation in patients with primary sclerosing cholangitis. J Hepatol. 1994;20:654–9.
77. Nichols JC, Gores GJ, LaRusso NF, Wiesner RH, Nagorney DM, Ritts RE. Diagnostic role of serum Ca 19-9 for cholangiocarcinoma in patients with primary sclerosing cholangitis. Mayo Clin Proc. 1993;68:874–9.
78. Ramage JK, Donaghy A, Farrant JM, Iorns R, Williams R. Serum tumor markers for the diagnosis of cholangiocarcinoma in primary sclerosing cholangitis. Gastroenterology. 1995;108:865–9.
79. Albert MB, Steinberg WM, Henry JP. Elevated serum levels of tumor marker CA 19-9 in acute cholangitis. Dig Dis Sci. 1988;33:1223–5.

2
Histopathology of primary sclerosing cholangitis

J. LUDWIG

INTRODUCTION

The gold standard for the diagnosis of primary sclerosing cholangitis (PSC) comprises the cholangiographic features of the disease[1]. They are described in this book by Dr E. Schrumpf. Despite the importance of imaging studies for the diagnosis and management of PSC, the expert analysis of liver biopsy specimens can also provide major diagnostic insights, primarily (1) in cases with equivocal cholangiographic findings, (2) for the diagnosis of possible complicating or associated conditions such as cholangiocellular carcinoma or autoimmune hepatitis[2], and (3) for the staging of the disease. Before the histological features of PSC can be appreciated, the general concepts of biliary disease classification – described in subsequent paragraphs – should be noted.

THE CONCEPT OF SMALL-DUCT AND LARGE-DUCT BILIARY DISEASES

Biliary disorders can be subdivided anatomically into large-duct diseases and small-duct diseases. The former are usually diagnosed by cholangiography and the latter by biopsy examination; prototypes for these conditions are choledocholithiasis and primary biliary cirrhosis (PBC), respectively.

As stated, PBC is the best-known example of a small-duct disease; indeed, the concept of a disease group with this name has emerged from the study of PBC, a disease in which microscopic bile ducts (interlobular and adjacent septal bile ducts) are destroyed while large, cholangiographically identifiable bile ducts remain essentially unaffected. In recent years many additional small-duct diseases have been identified – for example, rejection cholangitis in hepatic allografts, drug-induced cholangitis, and idiopathic adulthood ductopenia. The nonsuppurative destructive cholangitis that characterizes all small-duct biliary diseases affects the aforementioned microscopic bile ducts only; the process often leads to loss of most or even all bile ducts in this size range (ductopenia).

After duct destruction has advanced past a hitherto-undefined critical point, inevitable consequences ensue, primarily biliary fibrosis and cirrhosis with portal hypertension. Without liver transplantation these conditions usually end in hepatic failure.

In the past decade PSC has been increasingly recognized as another small-duct biliary disease; the major difference is that PSC *also* is a large-duct disease; in fact it is one of the best examples of a large-duct biliary disease[3]. The small-duct component of PSC was recognized long ago under the now-obsolete name 'pericholangitis'. Authors at the time had not clearly appreciated that 'pericholangitis' is the microscopic manifestation of PSC. Indeed, we now know that damage at the microscopic level primarily determines the progression of the disease, because this damage is the cause of the cirrhosis. The only exceptions are cholangiocarcinomas that may arise from large ducts in PSC and that may be fatal whether small-duct duct disease is present or not. In some instances the similarity between the biopsy manifestations of PSC and of PBC may be so great that even experienced pathologists cannot tell which is which.

LARGE-DUCT FEATURES OF PSC

Cholangiectases are a near-pathognomonic feature of PSC (Figure 1a–c). They can generally be appreciated only in large surgical specimens, native livers after transplantation, or autopsy livers. Study of such specimens clearly shows that the pruned-tree appearance of these ducts in cholangiograms is due to fibrous strictures and luminal obliteration. Biliary gravel or larger concrements, cholangitic abscesses, and tumours may be found associated with the cholangiectases in PSC. If ischaemic cholangitis and fibropolycystic liver diseases, such as Caroli's disease, can be ruled out, the large-duct lesions in PSC are diagnostic.

BIOPSY FEATURES AND STAGING CRITERIA OF PSC

In the early stages of the disease, biopsy findings may be essentially negative, or specimens may show only mild portal oedema, minimal portal inflammation, and some proliferation of ducts and ductules. Non-suppurative cholangitis may be noted (Figure 2) but the lesion lacks any diagnostic specificity. In a patient with inflammatory bowel disease – in particular, chronic ulcerative colitis – even minimal changes such as portal oedema and some ductal proliferation should raise a strong suspicion of early PSC. If ducts are proliferated in some portal tracts but appear absent in others, the likelihood that PSC is present is strengthened. Patients with these features generally have a cholestatic biochemical profile.

By and large, the progression of biopsy features in PSC closely resembles the changes observed in PBC[4,5]. Although both conditions are characterized by distinguishing hallmarks, such findings are not commonly seen in needle biopsy specimens of the liver. The near-diagnostic hallmark of PSC is the obliteration of small bile ducts, the end stage of fibrous–obliterative cholangitis (Figure 3a and b), whereas the hallmark of PBC is the florid duct lesion. In PSC, cross-sections of ducts that underwent fibrous–obliterative cholangitis resemble small nodules

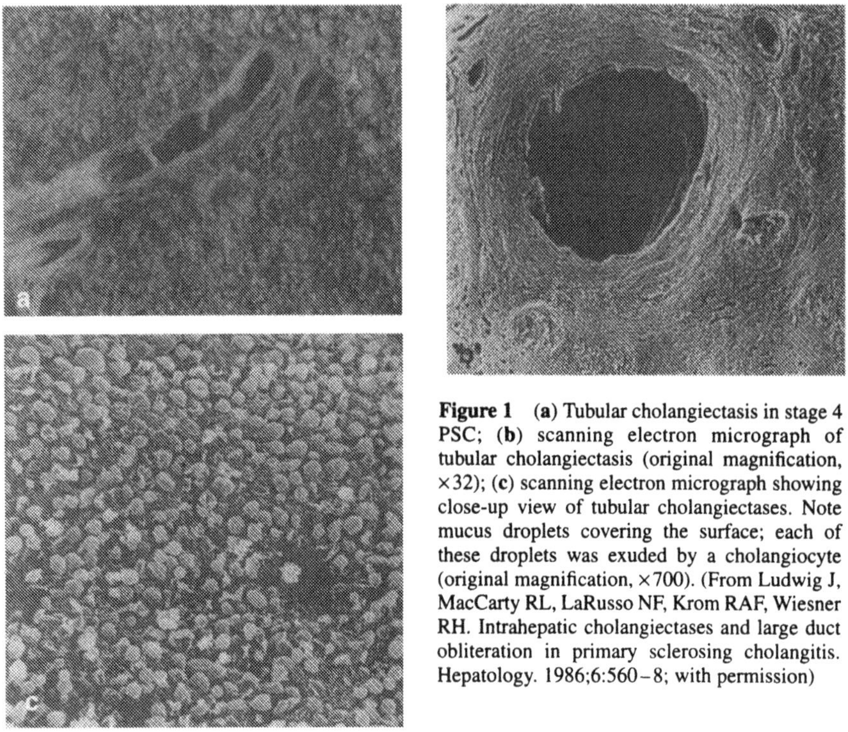

Figure 1 (**a**) Tubular cholangiectasis in stage 4 PSC; (**b**) scanning electron micrograph of tubular cholangiectasis (original magnification, ×32); (**c**) scanning electron micrograph showing close-up view of tubular cholangiectases. Note mucus droplets covering the surface; each of these droplets was exuded by a cholangiocyte (original magnification, ×700). (From Ludwig J, MacCarty RL, LaRusso NF, Krom RAF, Wiesner RH. Intrahepatic cholangiectases and large duct obliteration in primary sclerosing cholangitis. Hepatology. 1986;6:560–8; with permission)

of connective tissue (Figure 3b). These obliterated ducts can sometimes be found in wedge biopsy specimens, but they are exceedingly rare in needle biopsy samples.

The presence of granulomas and, in particular, granulomatous cholangitis, is generally considered a diagnostic feature of PBS and an exclusion criterion for PSC. However, granulomas may also occur in specimens from patients with PSC, although they are generally distant from bile ducts and almost never resemble true granulomatous cholangitis–that is, a classical florid duct lesion.

Another distinguishing feature of PSC and PBC are the inflammatory infiltrates which tend to be quite mild in PSC and may be severe in PBC. However, this finding is not reliable in individual cases. In the cirrhotic stage of PSC, biopsies usually reveal unequivocal biliary features; that is, garland-shaped regenerative nodules, cholate stasis, copper deposition, ductular and fibrous piecemeal necrosis, and ductopenia. In many instances Mallory bodies are present in the periphery of regenerative nodules, particularly in association with cholate stasis (this should not be misinterpreted as a sign of alcoholic liver disease!). Although these features are characteristic of biliary cirrhosis as opposed to cirrhosis following viral hepatitis, to name one example, they generally do not allow clear identification of the type of the underlying biliary disease. The four stages of the liver disease in PSC are schematically shown in Figure 4; the corresponding staging criteria are listed in Table 1.

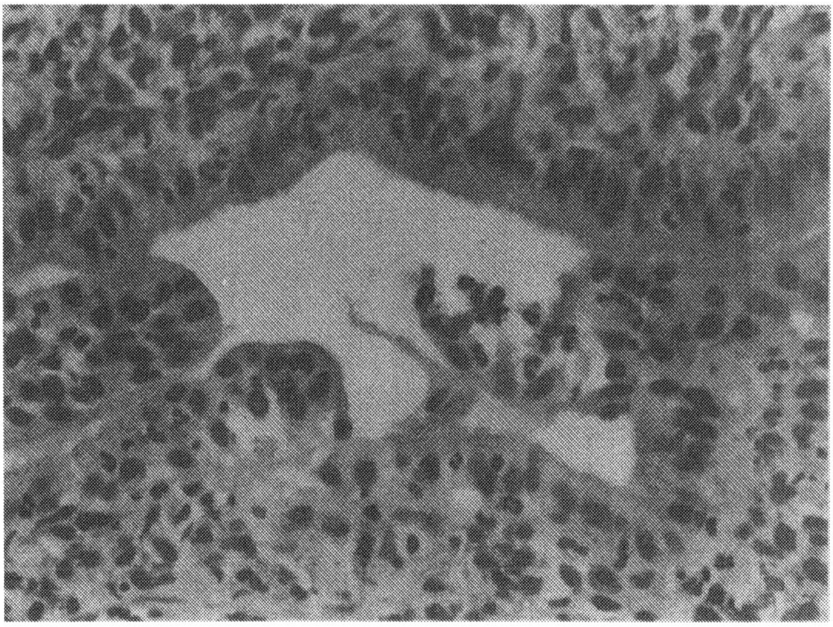

Figure 2 Non-suppurative cholangitis in early stage PSC. (From Ludwig J. Surgical pathology of the syndrome of primary sclerosing cholangitis. Am J Surg Pathol. 1989;13:43–9; with permission)

It should be noted that the staging criteria for PSC describe abnormalities of portal tracts and of the liver parenchyma; they are *not* determined by large-duct abnormalities as they can be seen in cholangiograms. This is justified by the observation that the progression of the disease towards liver transplantation or death is determined primarily by the changes in the hepatic parenchyma, not by large-duct changes. Of course, if a bile duct adenocarcinoma (cholangiocarcinoma) or a cholangitic sepsis develops, a catastrophic short cut of this progression may be observed.

Lastly, clinicians should note that, for the evaluation of PSC, *liver* biopsies are recommended; biopsies of extrahepatic bile ducts are not suitable for the diagnosis of PSC; they are justified only to rule out the presence of a neoplasm. Thus, the common bile duct in PSC is often chronically inflamed and scarred, but the very same features can be seen in other conditions[6] such as postoperative strictures and other manifestations of ischaemic cholangitis, as described in the next section.

PSC AND ISCHAEMIC CHOLANGITIS

Most biliary diseases involve either large or small ducts and only two conditions in these disease groups affect both duct systems with some regularity; one is PSC and the other is ischaemic cholangitis. This latter condition most commonly is found in hepatic allografts[7] after hepatic artery thrombosis or anastomotic

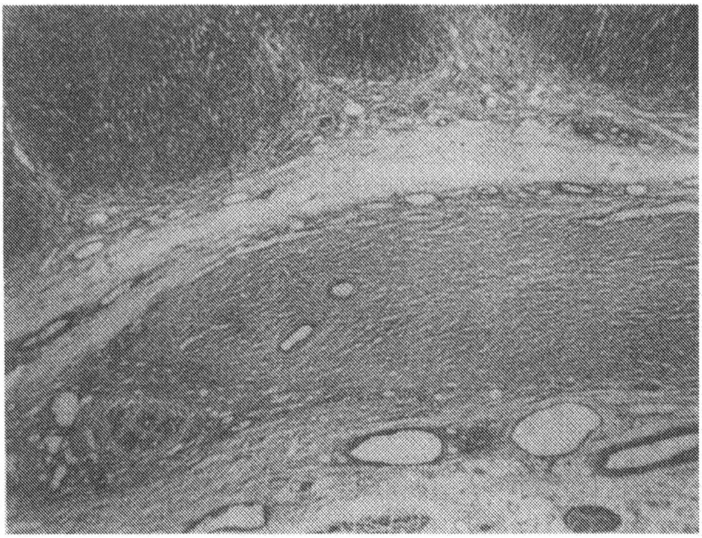

a

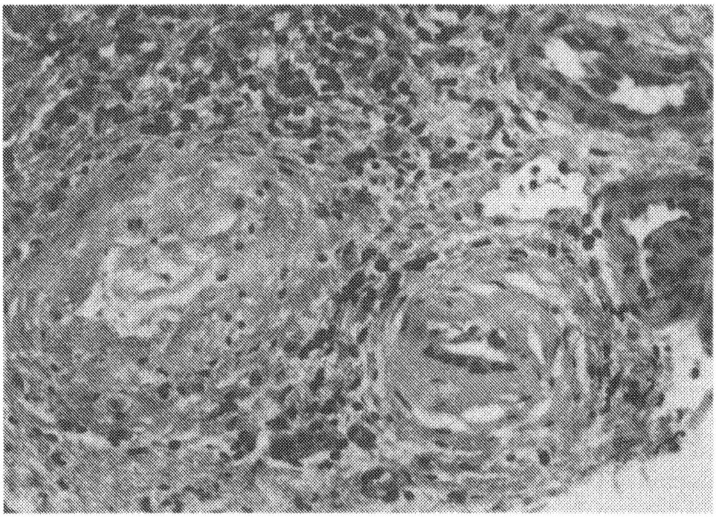

b

Figure 3 End-stage of PSC with duct obliteration. (**a**) Longitudinal section through obliterated duct in stage 4 PSC (From Ludwig J, MacCarty RL, LaRusso NF, Krom RAF, Wiesner RH. Intrahepatic cholangiectases and large duct obliteration in primary sclerosing cholangitis. Hepatology. 1986;6:560–8; with permission.); (**b**) biopsy features of duct obliteration in PSC. Note round scar on left and scar with remnant of epithelium on right. (H&E, ×125) (From Ludwig J, Barham SS, LaRusso NF, Elveback LR, Wiesner RH, McCall JT. Morphologic features of chronic hepatitis associated with primary sclerosing cholangitis and ulcerative colitis. Hepatology. 1981;1:632–40; with permission)

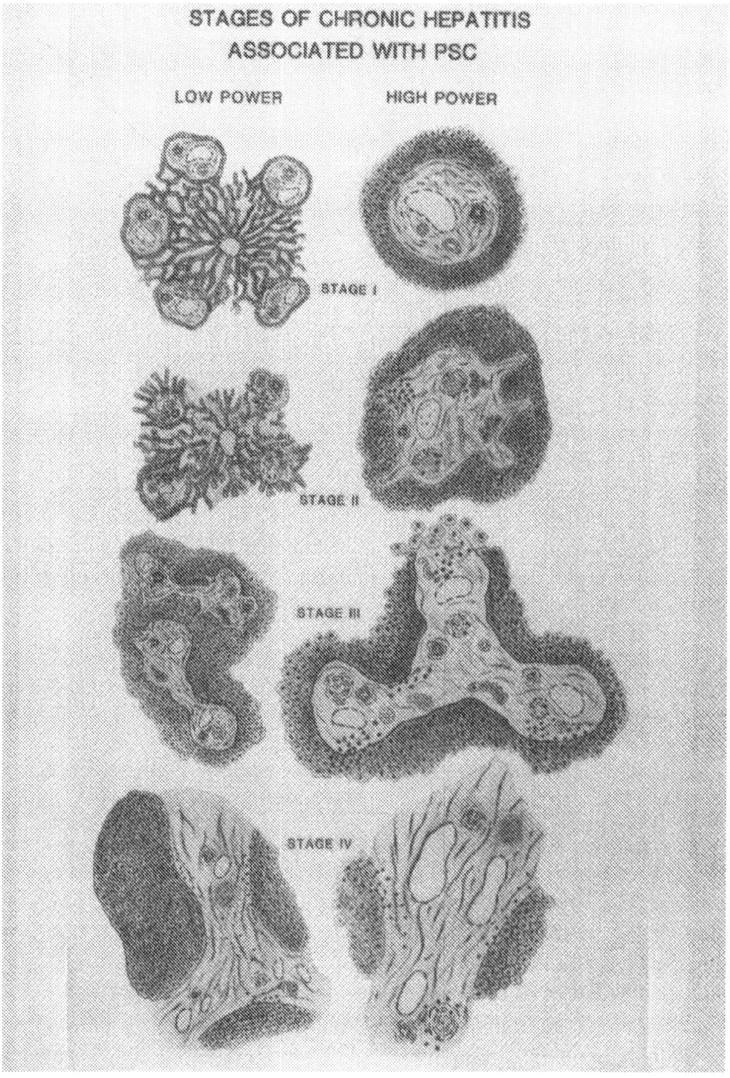

Figure 4 Stages of the chronic hepatitis in PSC. For a description of the features in the four stages, see text. (From Ludwig J. Surgical pathology of the syndrome of primary sclerosing cholangitis. Am J Surg Pathol. 1989;13:43–9; with permission)

stenosis and other causes of insufficient hepatic arterial perfusion or oxygenation. In the non-transplant setting, obliterative arteriopathy after intra-arterial floxuridine (FUDR) infusion has caused ischaemic cholangitis, but in rare instances perioperative mishaps have also been responsible for this condition[8]. The appearances of PSC and ischaemic cholangitis may be so similar that one might speculate that ischaemia also plays a role in the pathogenesis of PSC. Even

Table 1 The stages of the liver disease in primary sclerosing cholangitis

Stage 1: portal stage	Inflammation and duct abnormalities confined to portal tracts
Stage 2: periportal stage	Periportal areas (zone 1 of Rappaport) involved by inflammation, fibrosis, or ductular proliferation. Formation of new limiting plates may create appearance of portal enlargement
Stage 3: septal stage	Septal fibrosis or bridging necrosis can be identified
Stage 4: cirrhotic stage	Unequivocal biliary cirrhosis is present

From: Ludwig, Am J Surg Pathol. 1989;13:43–9

Table 2 Possible biopsy diagnoses in patients with primary sclerosing cholangitis in various clinical settings

Biopsy diagnosis	*Clinical setting*
Portal hepatitis with oedema and mild ductal proliferation (? incomplete obstruction)	Pathologist did not receive any clinical information
Portal hepatitis with oedema and mild ductal proliferation, compatible with stage 1 small-duct PSC	Pathologist was told that patient has chronic ulcerative colitis, a cholestatic biochemical profile, and a non-diagnostic cholangiogram
Periportal and septal fibrosis with ductular piecemeal necrosis and ductopenia, suggestive of stage 3 chronic biliary disease	Pathologist did not receive any clinical information
Periportal and septal fibrosis with ductular piecemeal necrosis and ductopenia, suggestive of stage 3 PSC	Pathologist was told that patient has chronic ulcerative colitis, a cholestatic biochemical profile, and a cholangiogram with features of PSC
Biliary cirrhosis (stage 4 disease) associated with PSC	Patient was known to have PSC; biopsy was done for staging purposes

if PSC is a primarily immunologically mediated disease, damage and incomplete perfusion of the peribiliary plexus could trigger a final common pathway and would make PSC comparable to ischaemic cholangitis.

The similarity between PSC and ischaemic cholangitis has made it extremely difficult to answer the important clinical question of whether PSC may recur after liver transplantation. Based on transplant experiences in general, one would expect that the disease indeed recurs, but some doubts persist because the cholangiographic features of PSC and of post-transplant ischaemic cholangitis are remarkably similar.

BIOPSY REPORTS AND CLINICAL DECISION MAKING

In order to allow for an optimal communication between pathologists and clinicians, efforts must be made to standardize the terminology and the format of the reports. Thus, terms such as 'pericholangitis' are as obsolete as the names chronic active hepatitis, chronic persistent hepatitis, or portal cirrhosis. We recommend strictly distinguishing between morphological and clinical diagnoses. Thus, names such as portal hepatitis, septal fibrosis, ductular proliferation, biliary piecemeal necrosis or granuloma are descriptive morphological terms that allow pathologists to record their morphological findings; these terms do not constitute clinical diagnoses! Since staging criteria (see below) are based solely on liver biopsy findings, the pathologist can often state the stage of the disease, but may be unable to say, for example, whether a patient has PBC or PSC. A few examples of biopsy diagnosis that might be expected in patients with PSC are listed in Table 2. The biopsy findings must be considered in the context of other test results and clinical findings. If this is done, diagnosis, prognosis, and therapeutic options can be readily established.

References

1. Lee Y-M, Kaplan MM. Primary sclerosing cholangitis. N Engl J Med. 1995;332:924–33.
2. Boberg KM, Fausa O, Haaland T *et al.* Features of autoimmune hepatitis in primary sclerosing cholangitis: an evaluation of 114 primary sclerosing cholangitis patients according to a scoring system for the diagnosis of autoimmune hepatitis. Hepatology. 1996;23:1369–76.
3. Ludwig J. Small-duct primary sclerosing cholangitis. Semin Liver Dis. 1991;11:11–17.
4. Harrison A, Hubscher S. The spectrum of bile duct lesions in end-stage primary sclerosing cholangitis. Histopathology. 1991;19:321–7.
5. Wiesner RH, LaRusso NF, Ludwig J *et al.* Comparison of the clinicopathologic features of primary sclerosing cholangitis and primary biliary cirrhosis. Gastroenterology. 1985;88:108–14.
6. Sherlock S. Pathogenesis of sclerosing cholangitis: the role of nonimmune factors. Semin Liver Dis. 1991;11:5–10.
7. Fisher A, Miller CM. Ischemic-type biliary strictures in liver allografts: the Achilles heel revisited? Hepatology. 1995;21:589–91.
8. Ludwig J, Kim CH, Wiesner RH *et al.* Floxuridine-induced sclerosing cholangitis: an ischemic cholangiopathy? Hepatology. 1989;9:215–18.

3
Immunogenetics and epidemiology of primary sclerosing cholangitis

P. T. DONALDSON

GENERAL INTRODUCTION

Primary sclerosing cholangitis (PSC) is one of three chronic liver diseases of putative autoimmune aetiology, yet neither the autoantigen nor the immune mechanism for the disease are known. One of the clearest indications that this may be an autoimmune disease is the observation of abnormal immune regulation in PSC and the well-characterized genetic association with particular HLA haplotypes, especially the 'autoimmune haplotype', A1-B8-DR3. However, even these 'facts' are based on observations from small patient groups and are subject to differing interpretations. In this chapter, I have attempted to review the epidemiology and immunogenetics of PSC in such a way that the manuscript is a self-contained unit. However, for the more discerning readers, I have included references to both original research publications and review articles. In writing this review, I have been critical of our own work and that of others, deliberately delving into current controversies, and, though I hope I have given a balanced account, some personal bias is inevitable.

EPIDEMIOLOGY OF PSC

Primary sclerosing cholangitis, a disease of unknown aetiology, is characterized by obliterative inflammation and fibrosis of the intra- and extrahepatic bile ducts. The diagnosis of PSC is based on the cholangiographic findings of strictures or irregularities in either the intra- or extrahepatic bile ducts (or both) in the absence of either choledocholithiasis, previous bile duct surgery, cholangiocarcinoma diagnosed or suspected 1–2 years prior to the presentation with PSC and acquired immune deficiency syndrome (AIDS).

PSC presents typically in early adulthood (25–40 years) though presentation in childhood is not uncommon. The estimated prevalence of PSC, based on studies of inflammatory bowel disease, is 1–6/100000. The majority of patients may have concurrent ulcerative colitis (66–100%) but the presence of inflammatory bowel disease does not correlate with liver histology. Deaths due to liver disease in PSC are from hepatocellular carcinoma, cholangiocarcinoma and complications of hepatic failure, including varices, encephalopathy and sepsis. Cholangiocarcinoma is detected in 6–9% of patients and other malignancies may occur, including lymphoma and carcinoma of the pancreas, prostate, colon and gallbladder. The prognosis is variable, with median survival estimates of 9–17 years. A number of studies have identified prognostic indices in PSC. In our own series, five factors at presentation were related to outcome: age, hepatomegaly, splenomegaly, serum alkaline phosphatase and histological stage[1].

There are few reports of familial cases of PSC and the best evidence of a genetic component to the disease comes from studies of the distribution of the HLA genes in population-based studies.

IMMUNOGENETICS OF PSC

Immunogenetics is a branch of science which brings together both immunology and genetics. In theory, this discipline encompasses all polypeptides with immune activity, though until recently immunogenetic studies have been limited to studies of the HLA genes (chromosome 6p21.3) and, to a much lesser extent, the other branches of the immunoglobulin supergene family, i.e. the T cell receptor (TCR, chromosomes 7 and 14), and immunoglobulin genes (Ig, chromosome 14). Interest in HLA and disease developed from early clinical studies of HLA matching for transplantation. The HLA system provided an ideal subject for genetic studies since there is very extensive germ-line (i.e. interindividual) polymorphism and both genotyping and phenotyping methods are easily accessed through an international network of transplantation centres. In contrast, TCR and Ig polymorphism which is mostly generated by somatic mutation and recombination, is more difficult and less frequently studied. Recently, investigators have turned their attention to a series of newly described genetic polymorphisms, relating various genes with immune function to disease susceptibility focussing on the cytokine genes in particular.

BACKGROUND

The genetic organization of the HLA region has been extensively described elsewhere and therefore I will discuss only those genes relevant to PSC. The HLA region spans approximately 4 million base-pairs of DNA on chromosome 6p21.3 (Figure 1)[2]. By convention, the region is divided into three subregions, HLA Class I (telomeric), HLA Class II (centromeric) and HLA Class III (located between Class I and Class II). The current WHO nomenclature for the HLA region is reviewed by Bodmer *et al.*[3] and the nomenclature of those HLA determinants referred to in the text of this chapter is summarized in Table 1.

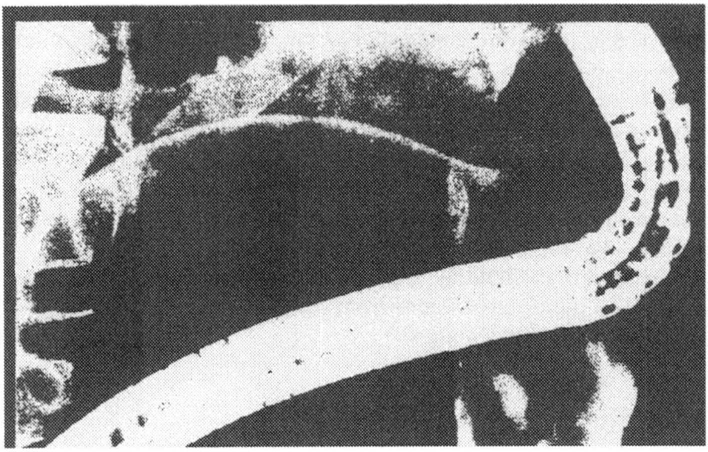

Figure 1 Human MHC (HLA region) chromosome 6p21.3. An abridged version of the human MHC gene map based on Campbell and Trowsdale[2]. Only expressed HLA genes are illustrated

Table 1 Nomenclature for HLA antigens and genotypes used in this chapter

Serological determinant		
Old name	*Current name*	*Allele**
HL-A1	A1	A*0101, A*0102
HL-A8	B8	B*0801, B*0802
HL-A12	B12	B*4402 to B*4406
Cw7	Cw7	C*0701 to C*0704
Dw2/Dw12[a]	DR2	DRB1*1501, DRB1*1502
Dw3[a]	DR3[b]	DRB1*03011,
DRB1*03012		
Dw4[a]	DR4	DRB1*0401
DRw6	DR13	DRB1*1301 to DRB1*1319
DRw6	DR14	DRB1*1401 to DRB1*1418
DRw52a/Dw24	DR52	DRB3*0101
DQ2/Dw3	DQ2	DQB1*0201
DQ3	DQ8	DQB1*0302

[a]Specificities determined by mixed lymphocyte reaction (MLR). [b]The common split of DR3 was called DRw17 later DR17; however, this term was not widely used before it was replaced by the designation DRB1*0301. *Current nomenclature is based on DNA sequencing data and is reviewed by Bodmer *et al.* (1997)[3]. In the current WHO nomenclature, the first four letters represent the HLA locus (e.g. DRB1) and the first two numbers following the asterisk give the broad allelic group, equivalent to the antigen defined by serology; thus DRB1*03 = DR3. The last two numbers represent the specific allele and are based on DNA sequencing data

HLA CLASS I GENETICS, STRUCTURE AND FUNCTION

There are currently more than one hundred genes or gene sequences mapped to the HLA Class I region. Of these, we are concerned with only three, HLA A, B, and Cw. These three transplantation antigens are highly polymorphic with at least 83 recognized alleles of HLA-A, 186 of HLA-B and 42 of HLA-C[3]. Each of these genes encodes a single polypeptide α-chain of 45 kDa which forms a non-covalent bond with a 12-kDa β_2-microglobulin molecule (the β-chain, encoded on chromosome 15).

HLA-A, -B and -C molecules are constitutively expressed on all nucleated cells though only weakly on hepatocytes. The expressed HLA Class I molecule is an α/β heterodimer spanning the plasma membrane with four extracellular domains, α_1, α_2 and α_3, from the α-chain and β_1 provided by β_2-microglobulin. These four domains make up a complex antigen receptor. The receptor site or 'antigen-binding groove' is formed by the α_1 and α_2 domains from a platform of crisscrossed β-pleated sheets surmounted by two opposing α-helices, one from each domain (α_1 and α_2). This closed-ended groove binds 8–9 amino acid polypeptides (antigens) derived from within the cell cytoplasm (endogenous antigen) for presentation to the TCR of CD8-positive T cells. The antigen-binding structure is supported by a stem provided by the α_3 and β_2 domains. HLA Class I–CD8 interaction is favoured by the presence of a CD8-binding site on the α_3 domain which helps to stabilize the HLA-peptide–TCR complex. Two other sets of HLA genes are required for antigen presentation by HLA Class I molecules. These are the TAP1/TAP2, and the LMP2/LMP7 genes. LMP2 and LMP7 are proteasome-β components which modify proteasome activity, whilst the TAP1 and TAP2 genes encode the transporter heterodimer known as the 'transporter associated with antigen processing' (TAP). During antigen processing for HLA Class I molecules, endogenous peptides are 'processed' into short peptide units of 8–9 amino acids by the large multifunctional protease or proteasome. Once processed, peptide is transported to the endoplasmic reticulum (ER) with the help of the TAP heterodimer. Once in the ER, the peptide may be bound by newly synthesized HLA Class I molecules. The TAP and LMP genes map within the HLA Class II region, and, though LMP is not thought to be polymorphic at present, there are five alleles of TAP1 and four alleles of TAP2.

HLA CLASS II GENETICS, STRUCTURE AND FUNCTION

The HLA Class II region encodes more than 30 genes, including genes which encode the classical 'transplantation antigens', HLA-DR, -DQ and -DP, as well as genes encoding TAP and LMP (above) and DM (DMA and DMB).

In contrast to HLA Class I, both the α- and β-polypeptides of the HLA Class II molecules are encoded on chromosome 6p21.3. Each of the DQ and DP subregions encodes a single pair of functional A genes and B genes, both of which have extensive polymorphism. At present, there are more than 18 alleles of DQA, 31 alleles of DQB, 10 alleles of DPA and 77 alleles of DPB. The DR subregion is more complex. There is a single, essentially invariant, DRA gene (encoding a 32-kDa α-chain) and 9 DRB genes, of which 5 are pseudogenes (DRB2, DRB6, DRB7, DRB8 and DRB9) and four (DRB1, DRB3, DRB4 and DRB5) may be expressed (each encoding a different 28-kDa β-chain). The number of DRB genes that each individual carries varies according to the DRB1 allelic group (Table 2) and is inherited as a discrete unit or haplotype from each parent. The DRB genes are highly polymorphic with more than 220 alleles listed at present.

HLA Class II molecules are constitutively expressed on specialized antigen-presenting cells, B-cells, monocytes, tissue macrophages, dendritic cells, endothelial and bile-duct epithelial cells but rarely on hepatocytes. The HLA

Table 2 Organization of the HLA-DRB genes in different haplotypes split according to the DRB1 genomic group. (Genes in italics are pseudogenes)

DRB1 allelic group	*Genomic organization*					
DRB1*01, DRB1*10	DRB1	*DRB6*			*DRB9*	DRA
DRB1*15, DRB1*16	DRB1	*DRB6*	DRB5		*DRB9*	DRA
DRB1*03, DRB1*11 DRB1*12, DRB1*13 DRB1*14	DRB1	*DRB*	DRB3		*DRB9*	DRA
DRB1*04, DRB1*07, DRB1*09	DRB1	*DRB7*	*DRB8*	DRB4	*DRB9*	DRA
DRB1*08	DRB1				*DRB9*	DRA

Class II molecule is expressed as an α/β heterodimer folded into four extracellular domains (α_1 and α_2, β_1 and β_2) and has a similar secondary structure to that of the HLA Class I molecule. In contrast to HLA Class I where the peptide-binding groove is an enclosed structure, the HLA Class II peptide-binding groove is open-ended, allowing binding of linear peptides of up to 24 amino acid residues. Antigenic peptides presented by HLA Class II molecules are derived from outside the cell (i.e. exogenous antigens) and are preferentially presented to the TCR of CD4-positive T cells. CD4–HLA binding is favoured by the presence of a CD4-binding site on the β_2 domain of the HLA Class II molecule. Exogenous antigens enter the cell through endocytosis and undergo proteolytic cleavage in acidic endosomes before binding newly assembled HLA Class II molecules which are then exported to the cell surface via the trans-Golgi. Antigen processing involves another HLA Class II heterodimer DM, the product of the HLA-DMA and -DMB genes. Newly synthesized Class II molecules are prevented from binding potential antigenic peptides indiscriminately by a molecular chaperone, the so-called invariant chain (Ii). The DM heterodimer performs the necessary function of enabling the invariant chain to dissociate from the HLA Class II molecule, thereby allowing peptides to access the antigen-binding groove.

HLA CLASS III GENETIC STRUCTURE AND FUNCTION

The HLA Class III region encodes more than 70 genes, amongst which there is a diverse array encoding immunologically active proteins, including the complement proteins C2, C4 (A and B), and factor B (Bf), tumour necrosis factor-α (TNFα) and lymphotoxin-α and β (LTα/TNFβ and LTβ), heat shock proteins (HSP-70, HSP-71, HSP-72) as well as a number of enzymes and pseudogenes.

The complement proteins, C2 and C4, are classical complement pathway polypeptides required for the conversion of C3 to C3d (C3-convertase) and C5 to C5d (C5 convertase). Factor B (Bf) has a similar catalytic function, combining with C3b to form a C3 convertase in the alternative complement pathway (Figure 2). There are two isotypes of C4, C4A and C4B, which may have differing affinities for amino and carboxyl groups. The genes from C2, C4A, C4B and Bf are all polymorphic. Abnormal complement function has been demonstrated in chronic liver diseases, including PSC[4,5] but whether this is secondary to liver damage is uncertain. Individuals with null or non-expressed complement genes

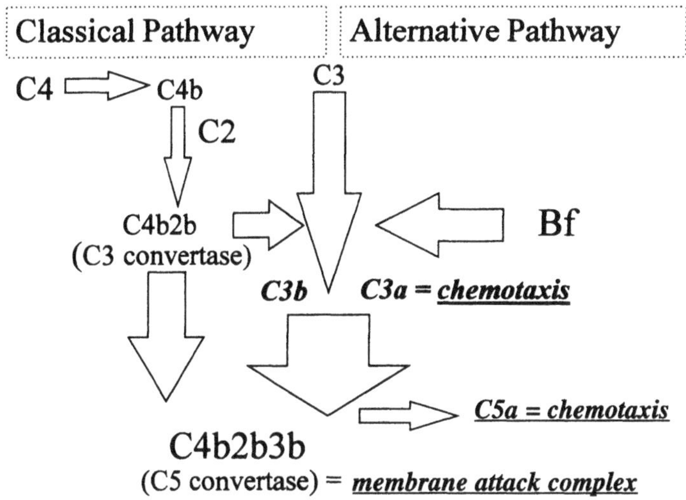

Figure 2 Functional relationships of the HLA Class III region-encoded complement proteins. Illustration of the HLA Class III complement C4, C2 and Bf gene function in conversion of C3 to C3b. C3b complexes with the C4b2b forming C4b2b3b (C5 convertase) which converts C5 to C5b, the first subunit in the membrane attack complex. C3a, the other C3 fragment, has weak chemotactic properties

(either deleted or otherwise) are more likely to develop lupus-like illness and homozygous C2 and C4 nulls can lead to complement deficiencies and may be lethal. Null alleles of C4A (C4AQ0) and deleted C4 genes have been associated with susceptibility to autoimmune hepatitis (AIH)[6,7] and primary biliary cirrhosis (PBC)[8,9] and though there are no studies of C4 and PSC, close linkage with the A1-B8-DR3 haplotype makes an association with C4AQ0 in PSC inevitable.

Tumour necrosis factor is a pro-inflammatory cytokine and an important mediator of inflammation and tissue damage in both autoimmune and infectious disease[10–12]. Although there is very extensive polymorphism of both the TNFα and LTα (TNFβ) genes (Figure 3), there is controversy over whether or not the described polymorphisms have any functional significance. Of particular importance here is the question of whether or not the two commonly studied TNF polymorphisms, TNF-308 and the NcoI restriction fragment of LTα, can be associated with low or high serum TNFα production[12]. An additional problem with TNF gene studies is the close linkage between HLA and TNF, particularly the A1-B8-DR3 haplotype which may hinder the interpretation of any associations described.

OTHER IMMUNOGENES IN PSC

Amongst the vast array of potential new immunogenes to investigate in PSC, two in particular are being extensively studied at present and both may be of particular relevance to our story. These are the IL-1 family (chromosome 2q13-

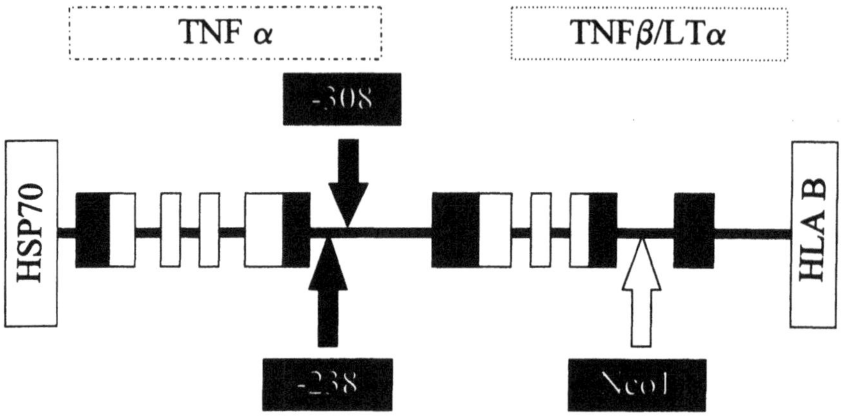

Figure 3 Illustration of the TNFα and TNFβ/LTα genes on chromosome 6p21.3 showing the positions of the commonly studied genetic polymorphisms −308, −238 and the NcoI RFLP polymorphism in the LTα region

14) and IL-10 (chromosome 1), both of which have limited polymorphism. The IL-1 gene family includes genes for the two agonist forms of IL-1, IL-1A which encodes IL-1α and IL-1B which encodes IL-1β, and the genes encoding the IL-1-receptor antagonist IL-1ra. There are two alleles of IL-1A and IL-1B whilst IL-1ra is marked by an 86-base-pair variable non-tandem repeat sequence (VNTR) with 5 alleles. It has been suggested that IL-1 gene polymorphism may be responsible for differential levels of IL-1 production and that this may be important in the pathogenesis of inflammatory diseases, including inflammatory bowel disease (IBD)[13,14]. This is of particular interest in relation to PSC because the majority (66–100%) of the patients with PSC may also have concurrent ulcerative colitis. Recent studies also suggest that IL-10 production may be low in PSC and PBC. This may be particularly interesting in light of recent evidence that genetic polymorphism in the IL-10 promoter genes may determine IL-10 production[15].

A PRACTICAL GUIDE TO HLA DISEASE ASSOCIATIONS

Understanding the significance of genetic associations with HLA

The first clinical studies of HLA and disease date from 1967 but even though some exceptional early studies identified very strong associations accounting for more than 90% of patients[16], it was clear from the beginning that most of the diseases being studied were not HLA linked. Notable exceptions include hereditary haemochromatosis[17,18] and congenital adrenal hyperplasia due to 21-hydroxylase deficiency[19]. Despite this, the general trend in HLA-disease-association studies has been to seek ever stronger genetic associations. Today few authors expect to find genes on the short arm of chromosome 6 or associations which approach 100% and it is now generally realized that these associations are, in most instances, part of a multifactorial/polygenic jigsaw[20].

Immunogenetics is mostly about comparing genes between disease and control populations (i.e. population genetics). The observation that a gene is present at a significantly different frequency in patients with a defined disease implies that the gene or a closely linked gene confers a degree of susceptibility (where there is an increased frequency) or resistance (where there is a reduced frequency) to disease.

The observation that the majority of genetic variability between HLA alleles results in amino acid substitutions within the antigen-binding groove has helped to promote a new era where HLA associations are described in terms of single or multiple amino acid sequences (motifs) at specific positions, rather than in terms of alleles or antigens. Substitution of one amino acid for another at a specific site may alter the antigen binding characteristics of the expressed HLA molecule, either directly through interaction with the antigenic peptide or through interaction with the peptide side-chains. The resulting conformational changes to the HLA–peptide complex may result in more or less efficient interaction with the TCR. These models are useful and may help to identify peptide-binding motifs of potential autoantigenic peptides, but these models are only hypotheses, are not necessarily correct in every case, and may over-simplify HLA-encoded disease susceptibility/resistance.

Linkage disequilibrium

Linkage disequilibrium is both a curse and a blessing for the immunogeneticists. Linkage disequilibrium occurs when there is non-random association of two genes encoded at different loci. Thus, when two HLA antigens occur together more often than predicted from their individual frequencies, they are said to be in linkage disequilibrium. The most prominent example of linkage disequilibrium is the HLA A1-Cw*0701-B8-DRB3*0101-DRB1*0301-DQA1*0501-DQB1*0201 haplotype, which is present in 12–16% of northern European populations but should occur in less than 1% of the population. Instead of being independently assorted, these genes pass from generation to generation *en bloc*, preventing an equal assortment or equilibrium. Though linkage disequilibrium is a problem in immunogenetics, linkage patterns can be useful, especially when comparing populations. For example: the haplotype DR4-DQB1*0301 has been associated with spontaneous (untreated) clearance of hepatitis C virus in Britain[21] whilst studies in France[22] identified DRB1*11-DQB1*0301. The similarities and differences between these two populations at a stroke provide strong suggestive evidence that spontaneous clearance of hepatitis C is associated with DQB1*0301 and that DR11 and DR4 are present only because of linkage disequilibrium. A full review of HLA associations in autoimmune and viral liver disease is published elsewhere[23].

Methods of HLA typing

In the data reviewed below, there are two eras of HLA typing, the era of serology (1982–1991), associated with poor-resolution HLA Class II typing and large-scale inaccuracies in antigen assignments, and the molecular era (1991 to the present), associated with high-resolution accurate genotyping.

Statistics

Statistical analysis is fundamental to practical immunogenetics and an excellent review was published by Svejgaard and Ryder in 1994[24] which includes a methodology for determining the strongest HLA association within a haplotype as well as determining linkage. It is important to briefly outline a few principles before we consider the data reviewed here.

HLA-disease-association studies are analysed using the χ^2 test and Fisher's exact probability test. Correction for multiple testing is essential, even in cases where there is an *a-priori* hypothesis (though the correction factor may be smaller). Comparison at 'the phenotype level' is preferred as counting genes effectively doubles the population without increasing the sample size and may lead to type II statistical errors. HLA-association studies often quote a value referred to as relative risk (RR) yet the value quoted in most cases is calculated from the cross-products ratio of the two-by-two contingency table and is in fact not the true relative risk, but a very crude approximation correctly referred to as the odds ratio (OR). Finally, it is common to see studies where secondary associations have been sought. This can be done by reanalysing the distribution of the HLA alleles after eliminating all patients and controls who possessed the first identified susceptibility/resistance allele (primary association). This practice allows the investigator to take into account bias introduced by a strong positive or strong primary negative association, thereby identifying hidden associations.

HLA AND PRIMARY SCLEROSING CHOLANGITIS

Early studies

Early studies of HLA and primary sclerosing cholangitis (PSC) described an increased frequency of HLA-B8 and DR3 in patients though HLA-A1 was not significantly increased[25–27]. These early reports based on small series of patients were published in 1982 and 1983. The first was a study of 20 patients from Oslo with 'ulcerative colitis combined with hepatobiliary disease'[25]. This was followed by studies of 25 patients from the Royal Free Hospital with well-defined disease[26] and a study of 16 patients from Oxford[27]. All of the patients studied were HLA-A and -B typed but DR typing was only performed in the Norwegian patients[25] and in 12 of the 16 patients from Oxford[27]. The first large series study, based on 81 patients from King's College Hospital, London, confirmed the HLA-B8 and DR3 associations and suggested that they may be due to an increased frequency of the A1-B8-DR3 haplotype which was found in 40% (32/81) of patients compared with 12% of 100 local controls[28]. The study also reported a strong negative association with the B44-DR4 haplotype and a secondary association with DR2. Though this study represents a landmark in PSC immunogenetics, with hind-sight, there is a number of problems. In particular, the use of serology in the assignment of the DR antigens may have resulted in an overestimate of DR3 and an underestimate of the frequency of DR6. Though similar criticisms can be made of most studies based on serological HLA-DR typing, this problem may be particularly important in PSC as we shall see.

The problem of using serology for DR typing was most clearly demonstrated by the study of Prochazka *et al.* (1990)[29]. In this series of 29 PSC patients, all 29 were found to have the DR52a serotype compared with an expected frequency of 35%. However, subsequent studies failed to confirm this extraordinary genetic association and eventually the data were withdrawn.

Recent studies

Following the Prochazka study, several centres set out to confirm the association using molecular genotyping. Three studies of HLA-DR[31–33], two of which included DQ[31,33] and only one study of HLA-DP[34] have been published so far. All three DR genotyping studies were based on PCR and included similar numbers of patients. The first study[31] was a single-centre study from King's College Hospital following on from the work of Donaldson *et al.* (1991)[28]. The positive association with DR3 (DRB1*0301) and negative association with DR4 (DRB1*04) were confirmed and a second susceptibility haplotype, DRB3*0101-DRB1*1301-DQA1*0103-DQB1*0603, was identified for the first time. It is an interesting detail of these two studies that the frequency of the DRB1*0301 allele was 12% lower in this series compared with the serological typed series[28] whilst the frequency of the DR6 allele DRB1*1301 was 9% higher. The underassignment of DR6 may have masked this effect in the previous study and the overassignment of DR3 may have introduced undue bias into the interpretation of future studies. The analysis of Farrant's study suggested that, because the two susceptibility haplotypes, A1-B8-DRB3*0101-DRB1*0301-DQA1*0501-DQB1*0201 and DRB3*0101-DRB1*1301-DQA1*0103-DQB1*0603, each encode DRB3*0101, then this must be the primary HLA association in PSC. Ironically, DRB3*0101 encodes DR52a. In addition, although the secondary association with DR2 (DRB1*1501) was weaker in this analysis than in the serological study the sharing of particular amino acid motifs by the DRB5*0101 (which is included in all DRB1*1501 haplotypes) and the DRB3*0101 alleles was used to create a model of susceptibility based on possession of a leucine residue at position 38 of the DRβ-polypeptide. Subsequently, the basic associations with the two susceptibility haplotypes and negative association with DRB1*04 (DR4) were confirmed by a study of the DRB1*0301, DRB1*1501, DRB1*12, DRB3*0101, DRB5*0101 and DRB1*04 allele frequencies in 83 PSC patients from Oxford and Birmingham[32] and a second full DR-DQ genotyping study based on 75 patients from three hospitals in Sweden[33].

However, there the similarity ends and controversy over the interpretation of the data from these three series begins. The Oxford/Birmingham study largely supported the King's data and agreed with the proposal that DRB3*0101 may be the primary susceptibility allele in PSC but was ambiguous about leucine DRβ38. Neither of these ideas were supported by the Swedish group who argued that the association with DRB3*0101 is simply the result of linkage disequilibrium with DRB1*0301 and DRB1*1301 and that there is no foundation for the leucine DRβ38 hypothesis in their series.

A second controversy exists regarding DR4. All groups observed a significant reduction in the frequency of DR4 but only the King's group interpreted this negative association as evidence of a protective effect of this allele. The Swedish group proposed that the lower frequency of DR4 may simply be a counterbalance for the two strong positive associations described (i.e. with DRB1*0301 and DRB1*1301). The low frequency of DR4 observed by the Oxford/Birmingham group was explained by an apparent close relationship between DR4 and prognosis (see below).

There is very little difference between these three studies and, though it is not possible to select one study from the others in terms of quality, there is a number of problems with them. In particular, none of the three studies applied statistical correction to the analysis of alleles identified *a priori*. This is not the correct procedure in this case. The null-hypothesis in each case was based on the number of candidate alleles and therefore a limited correction factor must be applied to the resulting probability values for these alleles (i.e. $p_c = p \times$ the number of *a-priori* alleles). In the study from Sweden, gene frequencies were used in part of the calculations. This is also contrary to advice (see above). The data which were not presented in the Oxford study (because only a limited number of DR alleles were tested) would, with hind-sight, be as useful as the data which were presented, especially the frequency of the DRB1*1301 allele or the distribution of the DQA and DQB alleles.

As an academic exercise, I have reanalysed the data from these three studies, applying a correction factor of 5 (i.e. the number of *a-priori* alleles tested) to the original data. When correction is applied, the emphasis on particular DRB alleles changes (Table 3). In the two UK studies, DRB1*0301 is no longer significantly associated with PSC whilst the negative association with DRB1*04 (DR4) remains significant. The outcome for DRB3*0101 is more variable and reflects differences in the patient and control frequencies for this allele in the two UK studies. Considering the two UK studies in the light of this fresh analysis, the primary association cannot be DRB1*1301 or DRB1*1301 which is only associated with PSC as part of the DRB3*0101-DRB1*1301-DQA1*0103-DQB1*0603 haplotype. The data from Sweden are less altered by correction with the exception that the DRB1*0301 association appears to be considerably weaker than that for DRB1*1301 or DRB3*0101. The difference in DRB1*1301 frequencies in Sweden and the UK may offer a partial explanation for the variation in interpretation of the HLA associations in PSC (Table 3) but also present a novel means of deciding the argument. Since one means of determining the primary susceptibility allele is to compare and contrast different populations seeking common associations, the most likely candidate as primary association for PSC is DRB3*0101. However, there is now a body or evidence to suggest that B8 is the primary susceptibility allele in PSC and that the associations with DRB1*0301 and DRB3*0101 are simply due to linkage disequilibrium (Donaldson PT, unpublished observations, September 1997). This model is unpublished and does not explain the increased frequency of the DRB3*0101-DRB1*1301-DQA1*0103-DQB1*0603 haplotype observed in all three studies above.

Table 3 HLA association with PSC: recent PCR-based published studies only

		Patients		Controls		
Series	*Allele*	*n*	*%*	*n*	*%*	*p corrected*
King's[30]	DR4	12	17	26	38	0.024
	DRB1*0301	31	44	16	24	0.06
	DRB1*1301	17	24	7	10	0.17
	DRB3*0101	39	55	15	22	0.00036
	Leu β38	56	79	32	47	0.0005
	Total no.	71		68		
Oxford[31]	DR4	17	20	27	42	0.022
	DRB1*0301	33	40	14	22	0.11
	DRB1*1301[a]	–	–	–	–	–
	DRB3*0101	41	49	18	28	0.046
	Leu β38	65	78	32	50	0.0017
	Total no.	83		64		
Sweden[32]	DR4	11	15	92	37	0.0015
	DRB1*0301	25	33	43	17	0.013
	DRB1*1301	33	44	45	18	0.000019
	DRB3*0101	40	53	70	28	0.00024
	Leu β38	56	75	132	53	0.0039
	Total no.	75		250		
	Grand total	229		382		

Note that the values in this table have all been recalculated. Probability is represented as p_c with a correction factor of 5 based on the *a-priori* hypothesis that DR4, DRB1*0301, DRB1*1301, DRB3*0101, and leucine at position 38 of the DRβ-polypeptide are associated with susceptibility or resistance to PSC. [a]Figures only available for references 30 and 32

The fate of DR4 is more easy to decide, considering that DRB1*04 remains significantly decreased in all three studies, even in the two UK studies where DRB1*0301 is not significant, and also considering the apparent strength of this negative association with DR4 throughout Table 3, it is not reasonable to argue that this association is simply a counterbalance for the positive associations with other DRB alleles, especially DRB*10301 and DRB1*1301.

Two relatively little-studied HLA loci in PSC are Cw and DPB. Early studies did not include HLA Cw typing, because good-quality Cw typing sera were generally unavailable. However, Prochazka *et al.* (1990)[29] noted a very strong HLA-C association whereby 86% of patients had Cw7. At face value, this association is much stronger than any of the associations described above. However, Cw7 is more common in the general population than any of the DRB alleles above and recent retesting of the C allele frequencies using molecular genotyping did not corroborate Prochazka's data with respect to Cw7, suggesting instead that the C locus may mark the telomeric limit for mapping HLA-encoded susceptibility to PSC (Moloney *et al.*, manuscript submitted, 1997).

HLA-DPB alleles in PSC were investigated by Underhill *et al.* (1995)[34] from King's College Hospital. The study was essentially negative with two important observations: there was no significant association with any of the DPB1 alleles and the association with A1-B8-DRB3*0101-DRB1*0301-DQA1*0501-DQB1*0201 haplotype does not extend to the DPB region. This clearly indicates that the centromeric limit of susceptibility to PSC must lie closer to the DQ region. No other studies have investigated DP or Cw.

NON-HLA IMMUNOGENES IN PRIMARY SCLEROSING CHOLANGITIS

The published HLA associations with PSC account for 50–55% of patients for any one allele or 75–80% for leucine DRβ38. This leaves 20–50% of patients outside the model. There are many other polymorphic immune genes (immunogenes): of which several are potential susceptibility genes in PSC?

Overall, there are very few studies of other susceptibility loci in PSC. The HLA-encoded complement genes have not been studied, nor have the other Ig supergene family members, TCR and Ig. Recent interest at King's College Hospital has focussed on the HLA-encoded TNF polymorphism (6p21.3) and the non-HLA-encoded IL-1 gene family polymorphism (chromosome 2q13–14).

The TNF data are promising with particularly strong associations being described with one of the two TNFα promoter gene polymorphisms at position –308, the TNF2 allele, and a weaker association with one of the two TNFβ promoter region Nco1 restriction fragment length polymorphism alleles, TNFB1 (Bernal *et al.*, manuscript submitted). However, these associations may be secondary to linkage with B8.

IL-1 in contrast, is less interesting, despite a reasonable chance of significant findings; considering the association between ulcerative colitis and both IL-1B2 and IL-1ra2, no significant differences in allele or genotype distribution were found (Donaldson *et al.*, manuscript submitted, 1997).

CLINICAL CORRELATES IN BOTH HLA AND NON-HLA STUDIES

There are two interesting clinical questions. The first relates to the possible relationship between HLA alleles and clinical outcome in PSC and is reflected in the controversy described in the previous paragraphs. In contrast to published data[31,32], the Swedish experience[33] reveals that neither DR4, DRB1*0401, DRB1*0301 nor DRB3*0101 are associated with a poor prognosis in PSC and there is no correlation between age of onset and HLA-DR2 or -DR3, and recent data from King's College Hospital concur (Moloney *et al.*, manuscript submitted, 1997).

The second question is whether immunogenetic markers distinguish between patients with and without ulcerative colitis. The weight given to this question depends partly on whether or not you believe that all or only a proportion of PSC patients have UC. Overall, neither HLA nor any of the other markers studied distinguish patients with UC from those without. This is not surprising since the HLA associations described with UC are weak but is perhaps surprising in relation to IL-1.

DISCUSSION, SUMMARY AND DIRECTIONS FOR FUTURE STUDIES

However you interpret them, the HLA associations reviewed above suggest that these genes are not simply markers, by virtue of linkage disequilibrium, for an undiscovered *disease gene* in PSC. The pathogenesis of PSC is likely to be multifactorial, perhaps involving multiple genes and environmental factors. The alternatives to the *linked gene theory* are that, either the products of these susceptibility genes act directly in the development of the disease process, or these genes are markers of disease severity or both. At present, neither of these hypotheses is fulfilled since we have considerable doubt regarding the leucine DRβ38 model and can find no correlation between HLA and disease progression. It is, however, too early to disregard either possibility. There are simply too few studies to answer this question at present.

HLA-encoded susceptibility to PSC is determined by two haplotypes, A1-B8-DRB3*0101-DRB1*0301-DQA1*0501-DQB1*0201 and DRB3*0101-DRB1*1301-DQA1*0103-DQB1*0603 and resistance is determined by the DRB1*04 alleles. The HLA-DPB and Cw loci mark the boundaries of susceptibility within the HLA region. Currently, it seems unlikely that either DRB1*0301 or DRB1*1301 are the primary susceptibility alleles in this disease. Two possible explanations should be considered: either DRB3*0101 is the primary susceptibility allele, or susceptibility maps outside the DRB region closer to HLA-B or DQ even. At present, there is only one large series which has published HLA-A and HLA-B allele frequencies in PSC.

Future studies of the HLA region must consider HLA-B, and may choose to look at the Class III region, in particular TNF and complement. In addition to considering the role of immunogenes on chromosome 6, there is a vast amount of work to be done outside HLA, investigating cytokine, adhesion molecule and complement genes.

References

1. Farrant JM, Hayllar KM, Wilkinson M *et al.* Natural history and prognostic variables in primary sclerosing cholangitis. Gastroenterology. 1991;100:1710–17.
2. Campbell RD, Trowsdale J. A map of the human major histocompatibility complex. Immunol Today. 1997;18:43.
3. Bodmer JG, Marsh SGE, Albert ED *et al.* Nomenclature for factors of the HLA system, 1996. Tissue Antigens. 1997;49:297–321.
4. Senaldi G, Donaldson PT, Magrin S *et al.* Activation of the complement system in primary sclerosing cholangitis. Gastroenterology. 1989;97:1430–4.
5. Brinch T, Teisberg P, Schrumpf E, Akessom I. The in vivo metabolism of C3 in hepatobiliary disease associated with ulcerative colitis. Scand J Gastroenterol. 1982;17:523–7.
6. Vergani D, Wells L, Larcher VF *et al.* Genetically determined low C4: a predisposing factor to autoimmune chronic active hepatitis. Lancet. 1985;2:294–8.
7. Doherty DG, Underhill JA, Donaldson PT *et al.* Polymorphism in the human complement C4 genes and susceptibility to autoimmune hepatitis. Autoimmunity. 1994;18:243–9.
8. Briggs DC, Donaldson PT, Hayes P, Welsh KI, Williams R, Neuberger JM. A major histocompatibility complex class III allotype (C4B2) associated with primary biliary cirrhosis (PBC). Tissue Antigens. 1987;29:141–5.
9. Manns MP, Bremm A, Schneider PM *et al.* HLA DRw8 and complement C4 deficiency as risk factors in primary biliary cirrhosis. Gastroenterology. 1991;101:1367–73.
10. Wilson AG, di Giovine FS, Duff GW. Genetics of tumour necrosis factor-α in autoimmune, infectious and neoplastic diseases. J Inflamm. 1995;45:1–12.
11. Grove J, Daly AK, Bassendine MF, Day CP. Association of tumour necrosis factor promoter polymorphism with susceptibility to alcoholic steatohepatitis. Hepatology. 1997;26:143–6.
12. Wilson AG, Symons JA, McDowell TL, McDevitt HO, Duff WG. Effects of a polymorphism in the human tumor necrosis factor α promoter on transcriptional activation. Immunology. 1997;94: 3195–9.

13. Mansfield JC, Holden H, Tarlow JK *et al.* Novel genetic association between ulcerative colitis and the anti-inflammatory cytokine interleukin-1 receptor antagonist. Gastroenterology. 1994; 106:637–42.
14. Bioque G, Crusuis JBA, Koutroubakis K *et al.* Allelic polymorphism in IL-1β and IL-1 receptor antagonist (IL-1Ra) genes in inflammatory bowel disease. Clin Exp Immunol. 1995;102: 379–83.
15. Turner DM, Williams DM, Sankaran D, Lazarus M, Sinnott PJ, Hutchinson IV. An investigation of polymorphism in the interleukin-10 gene promoter. Eur J Immunogenet. 1997;24:1–8.
16. Brewerton DA, Caffrey M, Hart FD, James DCO, Nicholls A, Sturrock RD. Ankylosing spondylitis and HL-A 27. Lancet. 1973;1:904–7.
17. Simon M, Pawlotsky Y, Bourel M, Fauchet R, Genetet B. Hemochromatose idopathique: Maladie associee a l'antigene tissulaire HL-A 3. Nouv Presse Med. 1975;4:1432.
18. Feder JN, Gnirke A, Thomas W *et al.* A novel MHC class I-like gene is mutated in patients with hereditary haemochromatosis. Nature Genet. 1996;13:399–408.
19. Dupont B, Obersfield SE, Smithwick EM, Lee TD, Levine LS. Close genetic linkage between HLA and congenital adrenal hyperplasia (21-hydroxylase deficiency). Lancet. 1977;2:1309–12.
20. Todd JA, Bain SC. A practical approach to identification of susceptibility genes for IDDM. Diabetes. 1992;41:1029–34.
21. Cramp ME, Carucci P, Underhill J, Naoumov NV, Williams R, Donaldson PT. Association between HLA class II genotype and spontaneous clearance of HCV infection. J Hepatol. 1988 [in press].
22. Alaric L, Fort M, Izopet J *et al.* Genes of the major histocompatibility complex class II influence the outcome of hepatitis C virus infection. Gastroenterology. 1997;113:1675–81.
23. Donaldson PT. Immunogenetics in liver disease. In: Manns MP, ed. Gastroenterology and Liver Immunology. Baillières Clinical Gastroenterology. London: Baillière Tindall; 1996;533–49.
24. Svejgaard A, Ryder LP. HLA and disease associations: detecting the strongest association. Tissue Antigens. 1994;43:18–27.
25. Schrumpf E, Fausa O, Førre Ø, Dobloug JH, Ritland S, Thorsby E. HLA antigens and immunoregulatory T cells in ulcerative colitis associated with hepatobiliary disease. Scand J Gastroenterol. 1982;17:187–91.
26. Chapman RW, Varghese Z, Gaul R, Patel G, Kokinon N, Sherlock S. Association of primary sclerosing cholangitis with HLA-B8. Gut. 1983;24:38–41.
27. Shepherd HA, Selby WS, Chapman RWG *et al.* Ulcerative colitis and persistent liver dysfunction. Q J Med. 1983;52:503–13.
28. Donaldson PT, Farrant JM, Wilkinson ML, Hayllar K, Portmann BC, Williams R. Dual association of HLA DR2 and DR3 with primary sclerosing cholangitis. Hepatology. 1991;13:129–33.
29. Prochazka EJ, Terasaki PI, Park MS, Goldstein LI, Busuttil RW. Association of primary sclerosing cholangitis with HLA DRw52a. N Engl J Med. 1990;322:1842–4.
30. Park MS, Terasaki PI. Inability to attribute susceptibility to primary sclerosing cholangitis to specific amino acid positions of the DRw52a allele. N Engl J Med. 1991;325:1252.
31. Farrant JM, Doherty DG, Donaldson PT *et al.* Amino acid substitutions at position 38 of the DRβ polypeptide confer susceptibility and protection from primary sclerosing cholangitis. Hepatology. 1992;16:390–5.
32. Mehal WZ, Lo Y-MD, Wordsworth BP *et al.* HLA DR4 is a marker for rapid disease progression in primary sclerosing cholangitis. Gastroenterology. 1994;106:160–7.
33. Olerup O, Olsson R, Hultzcrantz R, Broome U. HLA-DR and HLA-DQ are not markers for rapid disease progression in primary sclerosing cholangitis. Gastroenterology. 1995;108:870–8.
34. Underhill JA, Donaldson PT, Manabe K, Doherty DG, Williams R. HLA DPB polymorphism in primary sclerosing cholangitis and primary biliary cirrhosis. Hepatology. 1995;21:959–62.

4
Aetiopathogenesis of primary sclerosing cholangitis

J. M. VIERLING

AETIOLOGY: AUTOIMMUNE AND NON-AUTOIMMUNE

The aetiology of idiopathic PSC has not been identified[1,2]. Associations with HLA haplotypes, autoantibodies and chronic ulcerative colitis (CUC) have led to the postulate that PSC is an autoimmune disease[1–3]. However, this postulate remains controversial since major differences exist between PSC and classical autoimmune diseases (Table 1).

Inflammatory bowel disease (IBD) is associated with PSC in >75% of cases, with CUC occurring in >95% and Crohn's disease in <5%[1]. The association with IBD has been viewed as circumstantial support for an 'autoimmune' pathogenesis in PSC. Recent studies of experimental animal models, especially 'knockout' mice with T cell receptor-α deficiency, indicate that intestinal bacteria and the immune response to bacterial antigens play primary roles in the pathogenesis of colitis and development of perinuclear antineutrophil cytoplasmic antibodies (pANCA)[4]. Thus, the role of bacteria (reviewed in Reference 1) and the immune responses of genetically susceptible individuals is now being reinvestigated as an alternative to the hypothesis that CUC and its autoantibodies are the result of immune responses to autoantigens.

Table 1 Comparative features of classic autoimmune diseases and primary sclerosing cholangitis

	Classic autoimmunity	*Primary sclerosing cholangitis*
Female bias	Yes	No
Age	Children and adults	Children and adults
Autoantibodies	Yes	Yes
Autoantibody epitopes	Diverse	Diverse
HLA associations	Class I and II	Class I, II, III
Associated autoimmune diseases	Yes but not IBD	IBD
Response to immunosuppression	Good	Poor

IBD, inflammatory bowel disease

Aetiological factors, including infection, toxicity, ischaemia and neoplasia, have been identified that cause histopathological and cholangiographic changes reminiscent of PSC[1,2,5]. These observations suggest that potentially diverse aetiological stimuli can trigger pathogenetic mechanisms resulting in PSC-like lesions[1,2,5]. Any lesions resulting in biliary obstruction are capable of initiating mechanisms[6] involved in secondary biliary fibrosis and cirrhosis (see below).

MICROSCOPIC AND MACROSCOPIC PATHOLOGY

To be plausible, a postulated pathogenetic mechanism in PSC must account for the diverse pathology involving: (1) small ducts alone; (b) small, medium and large intrahepatic ducts; and/or (c) extrahepatic ducts. The pancreatic duct is rarely involved, indicating that all ductular derivatives of the embryonic foregut are potential targets in PSC. Small duct involvement is detectable only microscopically, while stricturing of medium or large intrahepatic or extrahepatic ducts is macroscopically detectable by cholangiography. Microscopic lesions of small ducts consist of predominant periductular inflammation and fibrosis, resulting in progressive epithelial atrophy and ductopenia[7,8]. Rarely, lesions of non-suppurative destructive cholangitis are observed. Microscopic lesions of fibrosing obliterative cholangitis and laminar circumferential fibrosis are more often observed in medium intrahepatic ducts[8]. Lesions of large intrahepatic and extrahepatic ducts consist of inflammation, fibrosis, ulceration and cholangiectasia. This diversity of pathology, as well as development of cholangiocarcinoma in up to 10% of patients, must be explained for any theory of immunopathogenesis to be credible[1,2].

IMMUNOPATHOLOGY

Portal tract infiltrates[9] contain neutrophils and CD4 T cells with increased proportions of monocytes/macrophages and decreased proportions of natural killer (NK) cells compared with peripheral blood. Peribiliary CD8 T cells are infrequent in precirrhotic PSC but common in cirrhotic livers[10]. Thus, they are unlikely to be primary effector cells, although they may play a role in the rare lesions of non-suppurative destructive cholangitis.

IMMUNOGENETICS

PSC is significantly associated with Class I, II and III HLA alleles[2,11] (Donaldson, Chapter 3). Molecular genotyping initially showed an increased frequency of two haplotypes: A1-B8-DRB3*0101-DRB1*0301-DQA1*0501-DQB1*0201 and DRB3*0101-DRB1*1301-DQA1*0103-DQB1*0603. A reduced frequency of DRB1*04 (DR4) was noted to correlate with less rapid disease progression. Reanalysis of genotyping (see Chapter 3) showed that the strongest associations were with HLA B8 and the Class III TNF A2 allele, while DRB1*1301 was not associated with PSC. The increased frequency of the haplotype DRB3*0101-DRB1*1301-DQA1*0103-DQB1*0603 was reassigned to the DQA1*0103-DQB1*0603 alleles, and the negative association of DR4 was extended to a haplotype including DQB1*0302. With respect to pathogenesis, it is noteworthy that HLA DR3 is associated with high TNFα production[12], possibly due to linkage disequilibrium with Class III TNF alleles[13].

AUTOANTIBODIES

PSC is associated with a variety of autoantibodies (Table 2). Between 70% and 84% of patients with PSC and CUC have pANCA[2]. pANCA, however, are not disease specific since they occur in high titre in the majority of patients with type 1 autoimmune hepatitis[14] and a minority of patients with primary biliary cirrhosis[15]. The specific antigens recognized by pANCA in each disease remain poorly defined. However, DNase digestion of neutrophils resulted in loss of recognition by CUC-associated pANCA while the majority of patients with PSC and type 1 autoimmune hepatitis exhibited a cytoplasmic ANCA reaction[16]. Evidence that the immune response of 'knockout' mice with T cell receptor-α deficiency to bacterial antigens results in colitis and development of pANCA[4] suggests that the pANCA in PSC may also be induced by responses to bacteria. Indeed, 81% of PSC patients (see Hopf, Chapter 5) have antibodies that react against enterobacterial proteins. The prevalence of anti-colon autoantibodies in patients with PSC and CUC is 62% compared with 17% in patients with CUC alone[17]. These autoantibodies do not cross-react with hepatobiliary tissue, while others reacting with epitopes of a 40-kDa molecule on colonic epithelial cells cross-react with antigens in skin and biliary epithelial cells (BEC)[18].

IMMUNOLOGICAL MECHANISMS OF BILE DUCT INJURY IN PSC

The immunopathogenetic mechanisms responsible for the variable microscopic and macroscopic pathology of PSC remain unknown. Although numerous immunological abnormalities have been described in PSC, their role in pathogenesis is unproved[2,11]. These abnormalities include: (a) decreased proportions of circulating T cells and CD8 T cells; (b) increased proportions of circulating B cells; (c) decreased T suppressor cell function *in vitro*; (d) increased autologous mixed lymphocyte reactivity *in vitro*; (e) immune-complex-like substances in blood and bile; (f) increased levels of C3b and C4d; and (g) decreased *in-vivo* clearance of artificial immune complexes by the hepatic macrophages.

Table 2 Autoantibodies in primary sclerosing cholangitis

Antibody	*Prevalence*
pANCA	70–84%
ANA	35% adults
SMA	55%
Anticolon	62%
Anticolon protein, Mr 40 kDa	67%
Antiendothelial cell	35%

Oligoclonal T cell receptor repertoire in PSC

Recent studies indicate that the hepatic T cells in PSC preferentially have Vβ3 T cell receptors (TCR)[19]. In contrast, no preferential TCR usage was observed in the peripheral blood. No correlation was noted with histopathological stage of disease. In another study, three cell lines were established from common bile ducts: two from PSC patients and one from a normal control[20]. Oligoclonal TCR were noted in the PSC patients and in one patient was found to be persistent in a second specimen taken more than a year later. Both cell lines proliferated when exposed to cultured enterocytes and were cytotoxic for enterocyte cell lines. Together, these observations support the hypothesis that T cells in hepatobiliary infiltrates may have been activated by limited antigen(s) and may react against epithelial cells of gut derivation. Their role in pathogenesis, however, is problematic because BEC do not appear to be targets of T effector cells in PSC[2,7,8].

Biliary epithelial cells as target cells

Recent studies have assessed whether BEC are targets of the immune response in PSC[2,11]. In PSC, BEC aberrantly express Class II HLA and ICAM-1 required for either presentation of biliary antigens to CD4 T cells or to be targets of CD4 or CD8 BEC-specific cytotoxic T cells. However, BEC are unlikely to play a direct role as antigen-presenting cells because they do not express the costimulatory B7.1/B7.2 molecules required for CD4 T cell activation[21]. Moreover, BEC do not concomitantly express both Class II HLA and ICAM-1 in PSC, indicating that only a minority of cells could present antigen or serve as targets of cytolysis[22]. The histopathology also argues against BEC as direct targets of T cells since NSDC lesions are rare and peribiliary CD8 T cells are infrequent in precirrhotic stages.

Inappropriate expression of ABO blood group antigens by BEC and colonocytes has been observed in PSC[23]. The cytoplasm of BEC from small and large bile ducts contained ABO antigens that were cross-reactive with anti-bile duct antibodies. There is no evidence of immunoglobulin-mediated duct injury or T cell reactions against ABO blood group antigens in PSC. Inappropriate expression may represent an epiphenomenon induced by cytokines or an early marker of dysplasia.

Endothelial cells of the peribiliary capillary plexus as target cells

The possibility that immune reactions could target the endothelial cells of the peribiliary capillaries in PSC is intriguing since it could result in ischaemic strictures and explain the atrophic appearance of biliary epithelia[7]. A recent immunohistochemical study of the peribiliary capillary plexus in PSC clearly showed that the capillary plexi remain intact in PSC but are pushed away from the bile duct by the peribiliary fibrosis[24]. Although it is unlikely that they are direct targets of immune reactions, the barrier to diffusion caused by periductular fibrosis may result in ischaemia.

Chemokines and cytokines

Both chemokines and cytokines may play important roles in portal inflammation, periductular fibrosis, atrophy of the biliary epithelia and extension of portal fibrosis. BEC produce a variety of chemokines and cytokines (Table 3). Cultures of normal human BEC and a cholangiocarcinoma cell line contain mRNA for the chemokine IL-8[25]. Secretion of IL-8 *in vitro* was stimulated by addition of recombinant IL-1β, TNFα or LPS (endotoxin), indicating that inflammatory cytokines or endotoxin may trigger BEC secretion *in vivo*. In contrast, BEC growth factors did not stimulate IL-8 secretion. Bile from PSC livers removed at transplantation contained significantly increased levels of IL-8 compared with bile from livers of patients with PBC, alcoholic cirrhosis or fulminant hepatic failure[25]. The BEC isolated from the PSC livers contained IL-8 mRNA and IL-8 protein was immunohistochemically detected in sections of ducts and isolated BEC. BEC also express the chemokine, monocyte chemotactic protein-1 (MCP-1). Attraction and activation of inflammatory cells by IL-8 and/or MCP-1 in the peribiliary environment could have diverse pathogenetic effects (Table 4). As noted above, the actions of chemokines may explain the characteristic composition of portal tract inflammatory infiltrates (neutrophils, CD4 T cells, increased monocyte/macrophages and decreased NK cells).

CD66a or biliary glycoprotein

Human bile contains CD66a, also known as biliary glycoprotein (BGP), which is a member of the carcinoembryonic antigen family and the human homologue of rat cell-CAM[26]. Neutrophils and monocytes express CD66 antigens that are involved in adhesion to E-selectin and act as receptors for lectins galectin 3 and bacterial type-1 fimbriae[26]. Specific crosslinking of neutrophil CD66a with CD66b or non-specific cross-reacting antigen 90 (CD66c) increases β_2-integrin-mediated adhesion and oxidant activity.

CD66a is also expressed in the canalicular membranes of hepatocytes, ductular epithelia, enterocytes and by some non-hepatic endothelial cells. In the human breast, CD66a is expressed in the apical domain of the epithelial cells and in myoepithelial cells[27]. Epithelial expression was decreased after development of malignancy, but remained intense in the myoepithelia in infiltrative radial scars and sclerosing adenosis. Although CD66a expression has not been characterized in PSC livers, its relationship to neutrophil function and myoepithelia in fibrotic lesions suggests a possible role in PSC pathogenesis.

Table 3 Expression of chemokines and cytokines by biliary epithelial cells

Chemokine expression	*Cytokine expression*
IL-8*	IFNγ
Monocyte chemotactic protein-1*	TGF-β_1 and TGF-β_2
	TNFα*
	IL-6*

*Not normally expressed; upregulated by inflammation

Table 4 Effects of chemokines

Target cells	*Actions*
Neutrophils	Neutrophil chemoattractant
Monocytes	$\uparrow$ intracellular $[Ca^{2+}]$
T cell blasts	$\uparrow$ exocytosis of granules
CD4 T cells	Upregulate integrins
Fibroblasts	Respiratory burst
Eosinophils	
Basophils	Monocyte stimulation
	Chemotaxis
	Upregulate integrins
	Respiratory burst
	Stimulate fibroblasts, T cells, eosinophils, basophils

Pathophysiology of biliary obstruction and cholestasis

Experimental bile duct obstruction results in a cascade of events[6]. The sequence of events includes: (a) increased LPS levels; (b) LPS activation of Kupffer cells and possibly portal tract macrophages; (c) secretion of IL-1β, TNFα, IL-6, TGF-α/β and leukotrienes; (d) TNFα-induced loosening of BEC tight junctions and regurgitation of bile; (e) LPS paralysis of BEC HCO_3^- production; (f) interruption of cholehepatic cycling between BEC and peribiliary capillaries; (g) BEC chemokine and cytokine secretion with recruitment and activation of neutrophils, monocytes and T cells; (h) enzymatic degradation of extracellular matrix; and (i) ductular proliferation. In rats with biliary obstruction, proliferating cholangiocytes secrete platelet-derived growth factor (PDGF)[28] that contributes to the cytokine activation of adjacent hepatic stellate cells. This fibroductular reaction can progress to secondary biliary fibrosis and cirrhosis unless obstruction is relieved. It is notable that PDGF is also expressed to a lesser extent by periductular mesenchymal cells and could activate peribiliary fibroblasts.

The pathogenetic mechanisms of biliary obstruction are pertinent to the pathogenesis of PSC. Both the microscopic and macroscopic lesions of PSC result in progressive obstruction and would be expected to trigger similar events. Thus, the key issue is the mechanism(s) that initiate the periductal inflammation and obliterative fibrosing cholangitis in PSC that secondarily stimulate the above cascade.

Animal models of PSC

Studies of animal models strongly suggest that the primary pathogenetic events in PSC may result from the immune response of an immunogenetically susceptible host to bacterial products of the gut. Two models, muramylpeptide-induced colitis in rabbits[29] and *Escherichia coli* chemotactic peptide-induced colitis in rats[30], are associated with histopathological lesions reminiscent of PSC. A rat model of small bowel bacterial overgrowth results in portal inflammation, bile ductular proliferation and cholangiographic stricturing of both intra- and extrahepatic bile ducts[31]. Pathology occurred only in a genetically susceptible strain and was not prevented by ursodeoxycholic acid, prednisone, methotrexate, cyclosporin A or polymixin B (which binds intraluminal LPS). Hepatobiliary injury was significantly correlated with TNFα production of Kupffer cells. TNFα production and hepatobiliary inflammation were prevented by: (a) mutanolysin, an enzyme that selectively cleaves bacterial wall peptidoglycan–polysaccharide; (b) palmitate blockade of hepatic macrophage phagocytosis; or (c) pentoxyphylline inhibition of TNFα secretion by hepatic macrophages. This model strongly implicates phagocytosis of bacterial cell wall components in portal venous blood by hepatic macrophages as the critical event. Moreover, the model is in accord with the recent observation that the immunogenetic predisposition to PSC is associated with the Class III HLA TNF A2 allele (see above).

Proposed mechanism of PSC pathogenesis

Based on the available data, the hypothetical pathogenetic mechanisms shown in Figure 1 are plausible. The critical initial event is postulated to be the reaction of an immunogenetically susceptible host to bacterial cell wall products resulting in TNFα production by hepatic macrophages and increased concentrations of endotoxin. Exposure to bacterial components would be increased by the presence of IBD but could also occur during episodes of gastroenteritis or bacterial

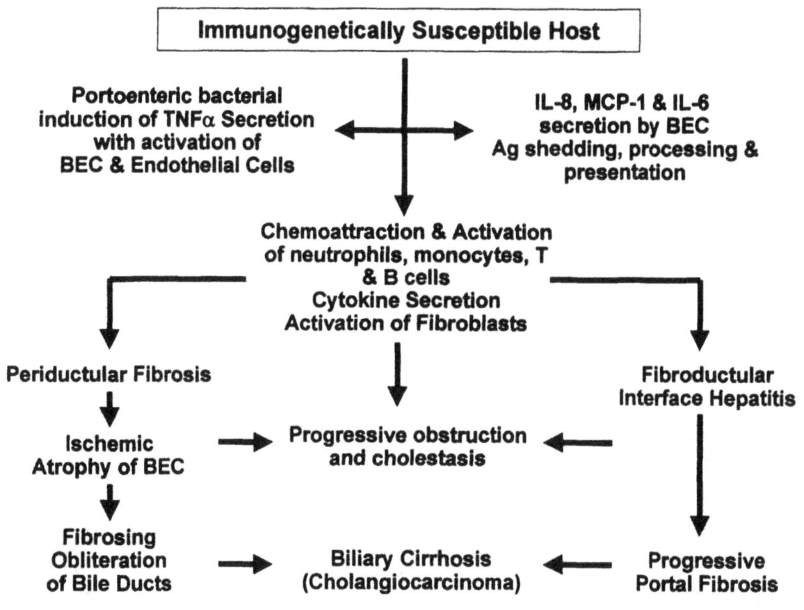

Figure 1 Hypothetical scheme of the pathogenesis of primary sclerosing cholangitis

overgrowth. TNFα and endotoxin in the peribiliary lymphatic space of Mall could induce BEC secretion of chemokines and cytokines, cause regurgitation of bile, interrupt the secretory function of BEC and the cholehepatic circulation. The peribiliary chemokine and cytokine milieu would favour attraction and activation of neutrophils, monocyte/macrophages, T cells and fibroblasts. Expression of PDGF by activated myofibroblasts would promote enzymatic digestion of extracellular matrix and deposition of peribiliary fibrous tissue. The expanding wave front of concentric fibrosis would push the peribiliary capillary plexi away from the bile duct, resulting in relative ischaemia associated with atrophy of the BEC. Progressive fibrosis would cause partial biliary obstruction and trigger the pathophysiological mechanisms of experimental obstruction. Further fibrosis would obliterate small bile ducts and severely stricture medium and large intra- and extrahepatic ducts, creating a vicious cycle of accelerated obstruction. Proliferation of cholangiocytes in the ductules would result in a fibroductular reaction with interface hepatitis, formation of bridging fibrous septa and secondary biliary cirrhosis. The combination of ischaemia, aberrant gene expression, altered local cytokine milieu and interruption of cholehepatic cycling may contribute to development of cholangiocarcinoma.

References

1. Vierling JM. Primary biliary cirrhosis. In Zakim D, Boyer TD, eds. Hepatology, 2nd edn. Philadelphia: W.B. Saunders Co., 1990:1158–205.
2. Vierling JM, Hu K-Q. Immunologic mechanisms of hepatobiliary injury. In Kaplowitz N, ed. Liver and Biliary Diseases, 2nd edn. Baltimore, Maryland: Williams & Wilkins; 1996:55–87.
3. Chapman RW. Role of immune factors in the pathogenesis of primary sclerosing cholangitis. Semin Liver Dis. 1991;11:1–4.
4. Mizoguchi E, Mizoguchi A, Chiba C *et al.* Antineutrophil cytoplasmic antibodies in T-cell receptor α-deficient mice with chronic colitis. Gastroenterology. 1997;113:1828–35.
5. Sherlock S. Pathogenesis of sclerosing cholangitis: The role of nonimmune factors. Semin Liver Dis. 1991;11:5–10.
6. Desmet V, Roskams T, Van Eyken P. Ductular reaction in the liver. Pathol Res Pract. 1995; 191:513–24.
7. Wee A, Ludwig J. Pericholangitis in chronic ulcerative colitis. Primary sclerosing cholangitis of the small bile ducts? Ann Intern Med. 1985;102:581–7.
8. Harrison RF, Hubscher SG. The spectrum of bile duct lesions in end-stage primary sclerosing cholangitis. Histopathology. 1991;19:321–7.
9. Hashimoto E, Lindor KD, Homburger HA *et al.* Immunohistochemical characterization of hepatic lymphocytes in primary biliary cirrhosis in comparison with primary sclerosing cholangitis and autoimmune chronic active hepatitis. Mayo Clinic Proc. 1993;68:1049–55.
10. Whiteside TL, Lasky S, Si L *et al.* Immunologic analysis of mononuclear cells in liver tissues and blood of patients with primary sclerosing cholangitis. Hepatology. 1985;5:468–75.
11. Freilich BL, Hu K-Q, Vierling JM. Immunopathogenesis of autoimmune hepatobiliary diseases. Curr Opin Gastroenterol. 1994;10:257–68.
12. Jacob CO. Tumor necrosis factor α in autoimmunity. Immunol Today. 1992;13:122–5.
13. Vassalli P. The pathophysiology of tumor necrosis factors. Annu Rev Immunol. 1992;10:411–52.
14. Targan SR, Landers C, Vidrich A *et al.* High-titer anti-neutrophil cytoplasmic antibodies in type 1 autoimmune hepatitis. Gastroenterology. 1995;108:1159–66.
15. Bansi D, Chapman R, Fleming K. Antineutrophil cytoplasmic antibodies in chronic liver diseases: prevalence, titer, specificity and IgG subclass. J Hepatol. 1996;24:581–6.
16. Vidrich A, Lee J, James E *et al.* Segregation of pANCA antigenic recognition by DNase treatment of neutrophils: Ulcerative colitis, type 1 autoimmune hepatitis, and primary sclerosing cholangitis. J Clin Immunol. 1995;15:293–9.

17. Mandal A, Dasgupta A, Jeffers L *et al.* Autoantibodies in sclerosing cholangitis against a shared peptide in biliary and colon epithelium. Gastroenterology. 1994;106:185–92.
18. Das KM, Vecchi M, Sakamakis S. Shared and unique epitope(s) on human colon, skin and biliary epithelium detected by monoclonal antibody. Gastroenterology. 1990;98:464–9.
19. Broome U, Grunewald J, Scheynius A *et al.* Preferential V beta3 usage by hepatic T lymphocytes in patients with primary sclerosing cholangitis. J Hepatol. 1997;26:527–34.
20. Probert CS, Christ AD, Saubermann LJ *et al.* Analysis of human common bile duct-associated T cells: evidence for oligoclonality, T cell clonal persistence, and epithelial cell recognition. J Immunol. 1997;158:1941–8.
21. Spengler U, Leifeld L, Braunschweigeer I *et al.* Anomalous expression of costimulatory molecules B7-1, B7-2 and CD28 in primary biliary cirrhosis. J Hepatol. 1997;26:31–6.
22. Broome U, Hultcrantz R, Scheynius A. Lack of concomitant expression of ICAM-1 and HLA-DR on bile duct cells from patients with primary sclerosing cholangitis and primary biliary cirrhosis. Scand J Gastroenterol. 1993;28:126–30.
23. Bloom S, Heryet A, Fleming K *et al.* Inappropriate expression of blood group antigens on biliary and colonic epithelia in primary sclerosing cholangitis. Gut. 1993;34:977–83.
24. Washington K, Clavien P-A, Killenber P. Peribiliary vascular plexus in primary sclerosing cholangitis and primary biliary cirrhosis. Hum Pathol. 1997;28:791–5.
25. Hiroki F, Matsumoto K, Melhem M *et al.* Participation of bile duct cells in biliary inflammation: production of IL-8 in response to irritant stimuli. [Submitted].
26. Stocks SC, Ruchaud-Sparagano MH, Kerr MA *et al.* CD66: role in the regulation of neutrophil effector function. Eur J Immunol. 1996;26:2924–32.
27. Riethdorf L, Lisboa BW, Henkel U *et al.* Differential expression of CD66a (BGP), a cell adhesion molecule of the carcinoembryonic antigen family, in benign, premalignant, and malignant lesions of the human mammary gland. J Histochem Cytochem. 1997;45:957–63.
28. Grappone C, Pinzani M, Parola M *et al.* Proliferating cholangiocytes contribute to liver fibrosis in the rat through platelet-derived growth factor expression. 1997 [Submitted].
29. Kuroe K, Haga Y, Funakoshi O *et al.* Pericholangitis in a rabbit colitis model induced by injection of muramyl dipeptide emulsified with a long-chain fatty acid. J Gastroenterol. 1996;31: 347–52.
30. Yamada S, Ishii M, Liang LS *et al.* Small duct cholangitis induced by *N*-formyl L-methionine L-leucine L-tyrosine in rats. J Gastroenterol. 1994;29:631–6.
31. Lichtman SN, Okoruwa EE, Keku J *et al.* Degradation of endogenous bacterial cell wall polymers by the muralytic enzyme mutanlysin prevents hepatobiliary injury in genetically susceptible rats with experimental intestinal bacterial overgrowth. J Clin Invest. 1992;90:1313–22.

5
Autoimmune markers in primary sclerosing cholangitis

U. HOPF, T. BERG, J. KÖRBER, R. KLEIN and P. A. BERG

INTRODUCTION

As a disease, primary sclerosing cholangitis (PSC) is a non-suppurative cholangitis which occurs in association with ulcerative colitis (UC) rather than Crohn's disease (CD)[1-11]. Usually, the inflammatory bowel disease precedes the effects on the liver. PSC may, however, persist for several years prior to the manifestation of bowel disease. The onset of PSC is of a chronic nature, and, mostly, with no substantial symptoms. Should there be an association with UC or CD, then the abdominal symptoms prevail. It is only with increasing cholestasis and cirrhotic evolution that those symptoms occur which can be partly attributed to liver disease, such as right upper quadrant abdominal pain, epigastric fullness, lassitude and possibly pruritus.

Secondary to microbial infection of the bile ducts and obstruction by gallstones, fever, jaundice, abdominal pain and biliary colics may occur in the early stages of cirrhosis. Polyarthralgia is frequent. At later stages, the development of icterus is a sign of already decompensated cirrhosis. With progression in time, PSC, as a predisposing disorder, increases the risk of cholangiocarcinoma.

The natural course of PSC is slowly progressive with intermittent recurrence of lesions. It may take 10–20 years for the biliary cirrhosis to lead to hepatic failure; this period may be shorter or longer. Due to the early onset of the disease, patients with fully developed cirrhosis who need liver transplantation are still relatively young.

In the early stage of PSC, alkaline phosphatase and γ-GT are increased. Histopathologically, a dense infiltrate of chronic inflammatory cells affecting bile ducts and portal vessels is characteristic. These lesions are progressive, leading, in the advanced stage, to expansion of periductal fibrosis and eventually to intra- and extrahepatic connective tissue scars with stenoses of bile ducts. Secondary to bacterial infection, a mixed morphological picture develops with signs of suppurative and non-suppurative cholangitis.

The aetiology of PSC remains unknown. As a cause, one could assume an intestinal trigger. The association of PSC with HLA-B8[5,12], HLA-DRw 52a[13] and

HLA-DR2 and DR3[14] suggests a genetic predisposition. The pathogenesis of PSC might be based on immunologically mediated processes, as indicated by the histological substrate as well as the detection of autoantibodies[15–18]. Further immunological findings show the presence of antibodies directed against intrahepatic bile duct epithelium which are cross-reactive to blood group antigens[19] and epithelium of the colon[20].

The diagnosis of PSC is established on anamnestic, clinical and laboratory grounds, but primarily on the results of ERC/MRC and liver histology. In the early stages, establishing the diagnosis may be cumbersome, since the typical alterations of the extrahepatic bile ducts as well as the characteristic morphological criteria of liver histology can be absent. The pathologist mainly detects histological features characteristic of a toxic hepatic alteration. A particular advantage in diagnosis at this stage is the detection of antigranulocyte antibodies (ANCA).

ANCA AND PSC

Serum autoantibodies reacting with the cytoplasm of human neutrophils in indirect immunofluorescence (cANCA) were described in patients with autoimmune vasculitis, and show a high degree of association with Wegener's granulomatosis[21]. An important target antigen of cANCA has been identified as proteinase 3.

The ANCA found in PSC show a perinuclear distribution pattern (pANCA). Data on frequency of pANCA in PSC vary between 40% and 90%[15–18]. These conflicting data may be attributed to different techniques used for the detection of pANCA[22,23]. Klein *et al.*[17] were able to identify positive pANCA antibodies in 87% of PSC patients after methanol fixation of the granulocyte preparations, whereas patients with UC without signs of PSC were positive for pANCA in only 17% of the cases (Table 1).

In a more recent study involving PSC patients at the Virchow Hospital, the same method yielded 89% positive cases (Table 2). The diagnosis was ascertained by ERC and liver histology. Using an ELISA test system with myeloperoxidase (MPO) as target antigen, the sera of less than 10% of these patients showed positive reactions while none were positive with proteinase 3, the target antigen of cANCA. We believe that, for routine diagnostic purposes, immunofluorescence methods should be used when PSC is suspected, while commercial ANCA–ELISA tests should be abandoned.

Recent studies show that the pANCA pattern corresponds to a range of distinct antigen–antibody systems which can be detected and differentiated by ELISA and immunoblotting methods[17,18,22–25]. Using granulocyte constituents as target antigens, several bands with molecular weights in the range 30–95 kDa could be detected[17,18]. Beside MPO, additional target antigens, such as bactericidal–permeability-increasing protein (BPI), azurocidin, cathepsin G, lactoferrin and others, have been identified[22–25].

Although highly associated with PSC, pANCA are not disease specific. Sera of patients with autoimmune hepatitis (AIH) show positive reactions in about 15%, and patients with primary biliary cirrhosis (PBC) are positive in 13–18%[17,18]. This holds also partly for patients with UC and CD.

Table 1 Frequency of antibodies to neutrophils (ANCA) detected by immunofluorescence and immunoblotting in patients with primary sclerosing cholangitis (PSC), primary biliary cirrhosis (PBC), autoimmune hepatitis (AIH) and ulcerative colitis (UC) (from Reference 17)

Diagnosis	*n*	*Immunofluorescence positive* (pattern)	*Immunoblot positive**
PSC	16	87% (80% pANCA)	80%
PBC	33	13% (pANCA)	11%
AIH	75	16% (p+cANCA)	13%
UC	23	17% (pANCA)	9%

*Bands at 30, 40, 55, 60 and 95 kDa

Table 2 Frequency of ANCA and other autoantibodies in patients with PSC and in the overlap syndrome of PSC with AIH

Diagnosis	*Positive for*				
	pANCA		*ANA*	*SMA*	*LKM1-Ab/LP-Ab*
	(IFL)	(ELISA) MPO as Ag	(IFL, IBL)	(IFL)	(IBL, CFT)
PSC (n=18)	16 (89%)	1	8	2	0
PSC+AIH (n=12)	11 (91%)	1	7	7	2/1

*Results from Virchow Hospital. Abbreviations: IFL, immunofluorescence; IBL, immunoblot; CFT, complement fixation test

Trigger mechanisms of ANCA as well as their pathogenetic importance are unknown. The frequent association of PSC with UC and to a lesser extent with CD, could suggest an enterobacterial genesis. This concept would be compatible with the fact that PSC–ANCA are mainly directed against components which play a role in immunological mechanisms involved in bacterial defence[26]. BPI of neutrophil cells, for instance, has high endotoxin-neutralizing activity and thus plays an important part in defence against Gram-negative bacteria. The induction of ANCA can be attributed to a peptide of human origin, e.g. BPI, which, after complexing with a lipopolysaccharide, becomes immunogenic. If the epitope of ANCA is also present in pathogens, molecular mimicry would seem possible.

OVERLAP BETWEEN PSC AND AUTOIMMUNE HEPATITIS (AIH)

An overlap between PSC and AIH is obviously more frequent than has been assumed up to now[27–29]. From the onset, PSC can exhibit additional markers of AIH. On the other hand, it may also take years before a manifestation of PSC engenders typical AIH criteria, and *vice versa*. An overlap between PSC and AIH should be taken into consideration when increasing levels of aminotransferases or high concentrations of IgG are present, and/or when autoantibodies typical for AIH, like, for instance, antinuclear antibodies (ANA), antismooth muscle antibodies (SMA), or antibodies against microsomal antigens (LKM-antibodies), or cytoplasmic antigens (LP- resp. SLA-antibodies), are present in high titres. In such instances, liver biopsy should be carried out. If the histological findings also include parenchymatous lesions, like periportal inflammatory infiltrates with piecemeal necrosis, then an overlap is sufficiently substantiated. This would have therapeutic implications, since, as would be expected, an immunosuppressive regimen is justified by AIH.

In a study with a cohort of 114 PSC patients, Boberg *et al.*[29] found a definitive overlap with AIH in 2%, and a probable overlap in 34% of cases, based on the AIH score of the International Autoimmune Hepatitis Group[30]. In our patients, including 30 PSC cases, 40% show a probable if not substantiated overlap with AIH (Table 2). ANCA are also found in AIH, although less frequently and not as exclusively as the pANCA pattern in immunofluorescence. Therefore, pANCA cannot be used as a differential diagnostic tool with respect to PSC and AIH[17,18,31].

The following case, originating from our 'Liver Ambulance Programme', demonstrates the transition from a juvenile AIH into a PSC resp. an overlap between AIH and PSC:

Patient D.L., female, was born in 1961. In 1974, she presented with LKM-antibody-positive AIH. Treatment with prednisolone and azathioprine led to remission of the liver disease. Between 1978 and 1986, sporadic elevation of ALT occurred with prompt response to prednisolone. In 1986, manifestations of UC began. In 1988, jaundice appeared: bilirubin 6.8 mg/dl, ALT 572 U/L, GGT 85 U/L, and alkaline phosphatase 251 U/L, albumin 3.2 g/dl, IgG 4343 mg/dl, prothrombin time 74%, thrombocytes 108/nl, LKM-ab positive, ANA 1:40, AMA negative, SMA positive, pANCA positive, and HLA-B8 positive. Liver histology: chronic aggressive hepatitis with cirrhosis. In 1991, cholestasis increased (alkaline phosphatase >1000 U/L) and decompensation of cirrhosis occurred. Prednisolone did not improve the liver disease; ERC: primary sclerosing cholangitis. In 1992, she had a liver transplant. Liver histology of the explant: cirrhosis with PSC (Figure 1). In 1998, she had normal function of the graft.

FURTHER SEROLOGICAL IMMUNOPHENOMENA IN PSC

In addition to pANCA, ANA are also found in PSC, with low or moderate titres in 40–60% of the cases. This phenomenon, however, seems to be inconsistent.

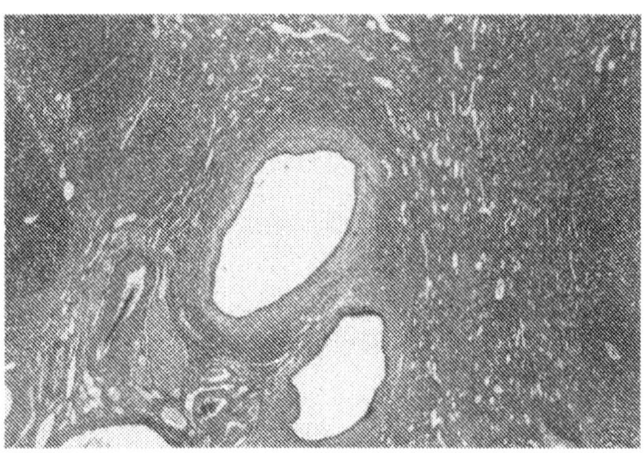

Figure 1 Explant of a patient with decompensated liver cirrhosis caused by autoimmune hepatitis overlapping with primary sclerosing cholangitis. The histology shows periductular fibrosis as well as parenchymal infiltration with piecemeal necrosis (× 150)

Strong elevated ANA titres can always imply an overlap with type 1 AIH; the same applies to smooth muscle antibodies (SMA) with antiactin specificity. The detection of LKM1- or LP-antibodies is consistent with the additional presence of type 2 or type 3 AIH. Antimitochondrial antibodies (AMA) are not found in PSC. An overlap between PSC and PBC is a rarity.

The immune response of PSC patients to Gram-negative bacteria has particular significance. Our own studies were able to demonstrate that patients presenting with PSC show antibody activity against proteins of enterobacteria, as shown by immunoblotting[32].

References

1. Thorpe ME, Scheuer PJ, Sherlock S. Primary sclerosing cholangitis, the biliary tree and ulcerative colitis. Gut. 1967;8:435–48.
2. Wiesner R, La Russo NF. Clinicopathologic features of the syndrome of primary sclerosing cholangitis. Gastroenterology. 1980;79:200–6.
3. Chapman RWG, Arborgh BAM, Rhodes JM *et al.* Primary sclerosing cholangitis: a review of its clinical features, cholangiography, and hepatic histology. Gut. 1980; 21:870–7.
4. Schrumpf E, Fausa O, Kolmannskog F, Elgjo K, Ritland S, Elgjo E. Sclerosing cholangitis in ulcerative colitis. A follow-up study. Scand J Gastroenterol. 1982;17:33–9.
5. Hopf U, Riecken EO, Zeitz M *et al.* Immunologische Parameter bei Pericholangitis und primär sklerosierender Cholangitis mit und ohne Colitis ulcerosa: Dtsch Med Wschr. 1983;108: 1515–21.
6. Wiesner RH, Grambsch PM, Dickson ER *et al.* Primary sclerosing cholangitis: natural history, prognostic factors and survival analysis. Hepatology. 1989;10:430–6.
7. Chapman RW. The immunology of primary sclerosing cholangitis. Spring Semin Immunopathol. 1980;12:121–8.
8. Farrant JM, Hyallar KM, Wilkinson ML *et al.* Natural history and prognostic variables in primary sclerosing cholangitis. Gastroenterology. 1991;100:1710–17.
9. Olsson RÄ, Danielsson A, Jarnerot G *et al.* Prevalence of primary sclerosing cholangitis in patients with ulcerative colitis. Gastroenterology. 1991;100:1319–23.
10. Ludwig J, Barham SS, La Russo NF, Elveback LR, Wiesner RH, McCall JT. Morphologic features of chronic hepatitis associated with primary sclerosing cholangitis and chronic ulcerative colitis. Hepatology. 1981;1:632–40.
11. Marotta PJ, La Russo NF, Wiesner RH. Sclerosing cholangitis. Bailliére's Clin Gastroenterol. 1997;11:781–800.
12. Chapman RW, Varhese Z, Gaul R, Patel G, Kokinon N, Sherlock S. Association of primary sclerosing cholangitis with HLA-B8. Gut. 1983;24:38–41.
13. Prochazka EJ, Terasaki PJ, Park MS *et al* . Association of primary sclerosing cholangitis with HLA-DRw52a. N Engl J Med. 1990;332:1842–4.
14. Donaldson PT, Farrant JM, Wilkinson ML, Hayllar K, Portmann BC, Williams R. Dual association of HLA-DR2 and DR3 with primary sclerosing cholangitis. Hepatology. 1991;13:129–31.
15. Snook JA,Chapman RW, Fleming K, Jewell DP. Antineutrophil nuclear antibody in ulcerative colitis, Crohn's disease and primary sclerosing cholangitis. Clin Exp Immunol. 1989;76:30–3.
16. Duerr RH, Targan SR, Landers CL *et al.* Neutrophil cytoplasmatic antibodies: a link between primary sclerosing cholangitis and ulcerative colitis. Gastroenterology. 1991;100:1385–91.
17. Klein R, Eisenburg J, Weber P, Seibold F, Berg PA. Significance and specificity of antibodies to neutrophils detected by Western blotting for the serological diagnosis of primary sclerosing cholangitis. Hepatology. 1991;14:1147–52.
18. Orth T, Gerken G, Meyer zum Büschenfelde KH, Mayet W-J. Antineutrophile zytoplasmatische Antikörper (ANCA) sind wertvoll in der Differentialdiagnostik der autoimmunen Lebererkrankungen. Z Gastroenterol. 1997;35:849(Abstract).
19. Jeffrey GP, Swanson NR, Yarred LJ, Reed WD. Bile duct antibodies crossreacting with blood group antigens in primary sclerosing cholangitis. Gut. 1990;31:698–701.
20. Das KM, Vecchi V, Sakamaki S. A shaved and unique epitope(s) on human colon, skin, and

biliary epithelium detected by monoclonal antibodies. Gastroenterology. 1990;98:464–96.
21. Gross WL, Csernok E. Antineutrophil cytoplasmatic autoantibodies (ANCA): immunodiagnostic and pathophysiological aspects in vasculitis. Curr Opin Rheumatol. 1995;7:11.
22. Wang G, Csernok E, de Groot K, Gross WL. Comparison of eight commercial kits for quantitation of antineutrophil cytoplasmic antibodies (ANCA). J Immunol Meth. 1997;208:203–11.
23. Hagen EC, Andrassy K, Csernok E *et al.* The value of indirect immunofluorescent and solid phase techniques for ANCA detection: a report on the first phase of an international cooperative study of the standardization of ANCA assays. J Immunol Meth. 1993;159:1–16.
24. Halbwachs-Mecarelli L, Nusbaum P, Noel EH *et al.* Antineutrophil cytoplasmatic andibodies (ANCA) directed against cathepsin G in ulcerative colisis, Crohn's disease, and primary sclerosing cholangitis. Clin Exp Immunol. 1992;90:79–94.
25. Stoffel MP, Csernok E, Herzberg C, Johnston T, Carrol SF, Gross WL. Antineutrophil cytoplasmatic antibodies/(ANCA) directed against bacterial permeability increasing protein (BPI): a new seromarker for inflammatory bowel disease and associated disorder. Clin Exp Immunol. 1996; 104:54–9.
26. Gabay J, Scott RW, Campanelli D *et al.* Antibiotic proteins of human polymorphonuclear leukocytes. Proc Natl Acad Sci USA. 1989;86:5610–14.
27. Minuk GY, Sutherland LR, Pappas SC, Kelley JK, Martin SE. Autoimmune chronic active hepatitis (lupoid hepatitis) and primary sclerosing cholangitis in two young adult females. Can J Gastroenterol. 1988;2:22–7.
28. Rabinovitz M, Demetris AJ, Bou-Abboud CH, Van Thiel DH. Simultaneous occurrence of primary sclerosing cholangitis and autoimmune chronic active hepatitis in a patient with ulcerative colitis. Dig Dis Sci. 1992;37:1606–11.
29. Boberg KMB, Fausa O, Haaland T *et al.* Features of autoimmune hepatitis in primary sclerosing cholangitis: an evaluation of 114 primary sclerosing cholangitis patients according to a scoring system for the diagnosis of autoimmune hepatitis. Hepatology. 1996;23:1369–76.
30. Johnson PJ, McFarlane JG. Meeting report: International Autoimmune Hepatitis Group. Hepatology. 1993;18:998–1005.
31. Targon SR, Landers C, Vidrich A, Czaja AJ. High-titer antineutrophil cytoplasmatic antibodies in type-1 autoimmune hepatitis. Gastroenterology. 1995;108:1159–66.
32. Hopf U, Stemerowicz, Knigge O *et al.* Primär sklerosierende Cholangitis (PSC)-humorale Immunphänomene, pathogenetische Aspekte und therapeutische Möglichkeiten. Z Gastroenterol. 1993;31(Suppl. 2):106–10.

Section II
Natural history and associated diseases

6
The natural history of primary sclerosing cholangitis

R. W. CHAPMAN

Unlike primary biliary cirrhosis (PBC), the clinical course of primary sclerosing cholangitis (PSC) is characteristically variable and unpredictable for an individual patient. Although the underlying histological process of bile duct loss is similar to PBC, other variables such as obstruction from large duct strictures, the formation of brown pigment stones and sludge within the biliary system, together with the unpredictable development of cholangiocarcinoma all contribute to the difficulty of providing the prognosis for an individual patient with PSC.

Although there was controversy in the late 1980s as to whether PSC is a progressive disease[1], recent studies from the USA and Europe have clearly demonstrated that, for the most part, PSC is a progressive disease and is now the main cause of death for patients with ulcerative colitis[2,3]. However, the clinical course of the ulcerative colitis does not appear to affect the progression of PSC[3].

PRESENTATION OF DISEASE

The presentation of PSC is defined as the first symptom, sign or abnormal investigation consistent with the diagnosis of PSC. It can occur at any age from early childhood to old age, although the majority of patients present in the third, fourth and fifth decades. In all reported series to date, two thirds of patients are male, in contrast to most diseases which are considered to be immune mediated, in which there is a female predominance. Fatigue is a frequent complaint, being found in approximately 60% of cases at presentation[4]. Other common symptoms include right upper quadrant pain, pruritus and jaundice. However, over the last decade, an increasing number of patients have been diagnosed who are asymptomatic at presentation, i.e. no symptoms referable to the liver. The disorder in such cases is usually detected as a result of routine biochemical screening of patients with total ulcerative colitis. The most common biochemical abnormality is a persistently elevated serum alkaline phosphatase concentration. In a recent series from Sweden, 44 of the patients were asymptomatic at presentation[4] compared with only 10% in earlier series from the 1980s[5]. Despite the name of the disease, clinical bacterial cholangitis is rare and usually occurs after instrumentation, such as ERCP or reconstructive biliary surgery.

The most common physical sign found at the time of presentation is hepatomegaly in approximately 50% of patients. Splenomegaly has been reported in some studies to be present in 25% of patients[6]. The serum alkaline phosphatase is nearly always elevated, although levels can fluctuate and cases have been reported with consistently normal alkaline phosphatase in the presence of diffuse biliary disease. The commonest cholangiographic finding is of biliary beading and dilatation affecting the whole biliary tree[5]. Approximately 25% of patients have changes confined to the intrahepatic bile ducts with cholangiographically normal extrahepatic ducts[4].

The histological changes at first presentation reflect the great variation in disease severity. In the series from King's College Hospital London, approximately a quarter of the patients were at each histological stage, so that 21% of the patients were at stage IV (cirrhosis) at presentation[7]. Approximately two thirds of cases in most series from America and Northern Europe have inflammatory bowel disease[5–7]. Reports from Southern Europe[8] and Italy[9] show a lower prevalence of inflammatory bowel disease, at around 50%, but this may reflect that ulcerative colitis was not actively excluded in some patients, as colonoscopy was not performed in all cases.

SURVIVAL

There is uniformity in median survival in the large series of PSC patients. The three largest studies, from North America[6], Sweden[4] and the United Kingdom[7], have all shown an estimated median survival of 12 years in symptomatic patients. In an earlier study by Helzburg *et al.*[1], only 15% of 54 patients died and the proportion of patients surviving was so high that the authors could not produce an estimated median survival, but instead produced an estimated 9-year survival of 75%. However, a high proportion of patients (21%) in a study by this group were lost to follow-up compared with a much lower proportion of patients in the other series. Aadland *et al.* reported a median survival of 17 years in a series of patients with PSC, all of whom had inflammatory bowel disease[10]. The reason for this prolonged survival may be that the diagnosis of PSC in patients with ulcerative colitis is made at an earlier stage; other series included patients with PSC without colitis.

CAUSE OF DEATH

The most common cause of death is liver failure and/or variceal bleeding which occurs in approximately two thirds of patients. The overall frequency of cholangiocarcinoma varies from 6% to 30% in recent series. In the large series of 305 patients with PSC reported from Sweden, 26% of these patients died of cholangiocarcinoma which was diagnosed a mean of 32.5 months after diagnosis of

PSC[4] had been established. In the whole group of patients with a follow-up of more than 5 years, 16% developed cholangiocarcinoma. This figure may still be an underestimate as not all patients in the series had an autopsy. Amongst the 65 patients who had died and had an autopsy or liver transplant, 29% had cholangiocarcinoma. There are no apparent differences between patients who develop cholangiocarcinoma and those who do not with respect to sex, age at presentation, extra- or intrahepatic involvement of the biliary disease or associated inflammatory bowel disease. Abdominal pain at diagnosis is seen more often in patients who develop tumours, as is an elevated serum bilirubin. It has been suggested that patients who smoke are at greater danger of developing cholangiocarcinoma. No immunogenetic factors have been identified which predict the predisposition to cholangiocarcinoma.

It is well established in PSC that there is an increased prevalence of HLA antigens B8 and DR3[11] and a negative association with HLA DR4 has been found in most series[11]. Interestingly, recent studies have shown that the presence of HLA DR4 is associated with an adverse prognosis with a more rapid progression to death or transplantation[12]. This HLA antigen is associated with a worse prognosis in patients with rheumatoid arthritis, although the explanation for this finding is unclear.

The association between HLA DR4 and poor prognosis needs further confirmation, as not all studies have shown this finding[13].

NATURAL HISTORY OF ASYMPTOMATIC PATIENTS

Some reports have suggested that the presence of antineutrophil cytoplasmic antibodies is associated with an early onset of disease[14], but later studies have not confirmed this association[15]. The clinical course of asymptomatic PSC has been controversial following the original description of three patients with no symptoms of liver disease who remained well for up to 15 years after diagnosis[16]. Heltzberg *et al.*[1], reported 13 of 53 patients who were asymptomatic at presentation, and remained so during the mean follow-up period of 56 months. This was in contrast to the findings from the Mayo Clinic group, where 76% of 45 asymptomatic patients had clinical or laboratory evidence of disease progression during a median follow-up of 75 months; 31% of these patients developed liver failure, resulting in death or referral for liver transplantation[17]. Their findings were confirmed by King's College who followed 19 asymptomatic patients, more than half of whom developed symptoms during a 5-year follow-up period[7].

In the largest and most recent study reported, 134 (44%) of patients were asymptomatic at the time of diagnosis[4]. The survival rate for the asymptomatic group was 70% at 16 years after initial diagnosis. However, 22% of all asymptomatic patients developed symptoms during a median observation time of 69 months and approximately 13% of asymptomatic patients died or had liver transplantation during the follow-up period. This emphasizes that PSC is a progressive disease even in asymptomatic patients, although not all asymptomatic patients appear to progress.

Table 1 Independent variables associated with a poor prognosis in primary sclerosing cholangitis – obtained from four different models

Independent variable	*Models*			
	Mayo 1989[6]	*King's 1991*[7]	*Multicentre 1992*[18]	*Sweden 1996*[4]
Older age	Y	Y	Y	Y
Hepatomegaly	N	Y	N	N
Splenomegaly	N	Y	Y	N
Inflammatory bowel disease	Y	N	N	N
High bilirubin	Y	N	Y	Y
High alkaline phosphatase	N	Y	N	N
Low haemoglobin	N	N	N	N
Advanced histological stage	Y	Y	Y	Y

Y = positively associated; N = not associated

PROGNOSTIC MODELS

A number of studies have now looked at the prognosis of PSC using both univariate and multivariate analysis[4–6]. Univariate analysis identifies all features which are prognostically significant whereas in multivariate analysis only those features which affect prognosis independently of all the other factors are identified. Once identified, the prognostic factors from the multivariate analysis can be combined to produce a mathematical prognostic index. As with PBC, a number of centres have attempted to arrive at survival models based on the clinical biochemical, biochemical and histological features of disease[4,6,7,18] (Table 1). The Mayo Clinic group have derived a model, based on clinical data on 426 patients from 5 major liver centres throughout the world, using serum bilirubin level, histological stage, patient age and the presence of splenomegaly as the significant prognostic variables[16]. In the more-recent Swedish study, it was found that age, serum bilirubin concentration and histological stage at the time of diagnosis were independent predictors of bad prognosis and these variables were used to construct a new prognostic model[4]. However, none of the models which have been published to date have been evaluated prospectively, nor cross-validated by other centres. Clearly, further studies are required in order to refine and increase the usefulness of prognostic modelling in PSC.

References

1. Helzberg JH, Petersen JM, Boyer JL. Improved survival with primary sclerosing cholangitis: a review of clinicopathologic features and comparison of symptomatic and asymptomatic patients. Gastroenterology. 1987;92:1869–75.
2. Olsson R, Danielsson A, Jarnerot G, Lindstrom E, Loof L, Rolny P. Prevalence of primary sclerosing cholangitis in patients with ulcerative colitis. Gastroenterology. 1991;100:1319–23.
3. Broome U, Galumann H, Hellers G, Sorstad J, Nilsson B, Hulterantz R. Liver disease in ulcerative colitis. An epidemiological and follow-up study in the country of Stockholm. Gut. 1994;35: 84–9.
4. Broome U, Olsson R, Loof L *et al.* Natural history and prognostic factors in 305 Swedish patients with PSC. Gut. 1996;38:610–15.

5. Chapman RWG, Arborgh BAM, Rhodes JM *et al.* Primary sclerosing cholangitis: a review of its clinical features, cholangiography and hepatic histology. Gut. 1980;21:1870–7.
6. Wiesner TH, Grambsch PB, Dickson ER *et al.* Primary sclerosing cholangitis: natural history, prognostic factors, and survival analysis. Hepatology. 1989;10:430–6.
7. Farrant JM, Hayllar KM, Wilkinson ML, Karani J, Portmann BC, Westaby D. Natural history and prognostic variables in primary sclerosing cholangitis. Gastroenterology. 1991;100: 1710–17.
8. Escorsell A, Pares A, Rodes J, Solis-Herruzo JA, Miras M, De la Morena E. Epidemiology of primary sclerosing cholangitis in Spain. J Hepatol. 1994;21:787–91.
9. Okolicsanyi L, Fabris L, Viaggi S, Carulli N, Podda M, Ricu G and the Italian PSC Group. Primary sclerosing cholangitis: clinical presentation, natural history and prognostic variables: an Italian multicentre study. Eur J Gastroenterol Hepatol. 1996;8:687–91.
10. Aadland E, Schrumpf E, Fausa O *et al.* Primary sclerosing cholangitis: a long-term follow-up study. Scand J Gastroenterol. 1987;22:655–64.
11. Donaldson PT, Farrant JM, Wilkinson ML, Hayllar K, Portman BC, Williams R. Dual association of HLA DR2 and DR3 with primary sclerosing cholangitis. Hepatology. 1991;13: 129–33.
12. Mehal WZ, Dennis Lo Y-M, Wordsworth BP *et al.* HLA DR4 is a marker for rapid disease progression in primary sclerosing cholangitis. Gastroenterology. 1994;106:160–7.
13. Olerup O, Olsson R, Hultcrantz R, Broome U. HLA-DR3 and DQ alleles are not markers for rapid disease progression in Swedish patients with primary sclerosing cholangitis. Gastroenterology. 1995;108:870–8.
14. Pokorny CS, Norton ID, McCaughan GW, Selby WS. Antineutrophil cytoplasmic antibody: a prognostic indicator in primary sclerosing cholangitis. J Gastroenterol Hepatol. 1994;9:40–4.
15. Mehal WZ, Lo SK, Chapman RWG, Fleming KA. The immunogenetic basis for antineutrophil cytoplasmic antibody production in primary sclerosing cholangitis and ulcerative colitis. J Hepatol. 1994;21:910–11.
16. Chapman RWG, Burroughs AK, Bass NM, Sherlock S. Longstanding asymptomatic primary sclerosing cholangitis: report of three cases. Dig Dis Sci. 1981;26:78–82.
17. Porayko MK, Wiesner RH, LaRusso NF *et al.* Patients with asymptomatic primary sclerosing cholangitis frequently have progressive disease. Gastroenterology. 1990;98:1594–602.
18. Dickson ER, Murtaugh PA, Wiesner RH *et al.* Primary sclerosing cholangitis: refinement and validation of survival models. Gastroenterology. 1992;103:1893–901.

7
Primary sclerosing cholangitis – relationship to inflammatory bowel disease

U. BROOMÉ

INTRODUCTION

The association between ulcerative colitis (UC) and liver disease was first recognized by Thomas in 1873[1]. During the late 1940s and early 1950s, numerous surveys of liver dysfunction in patients with UC were presented and it was concluded that the prevalence of liver disturbances in UC was higher than in the general population[2,3]. Hepatic disorders reported in association with UC included fatty change, chronic active hepatitis, cirrhosis, pericholangitis and cholangiocarcinoma. The association of primary sclerosing cholangitis (PSC) with UC was first shown in 1965 by Smith and Loe[4] and was subsequently confirmed by others[5]. A 25–30% incidence of IBD was noted in PSC patients. With the increased clinical awareness of the relationship between PSC and UC, patients with UC are more frequently screened with liver function tests. Furthermore, with the increased use of endoscopic retrograde cholangiography (ERCP), more patients with PSC are identified, especially among patients with inflammatory bowel disease (IBD), suggesting that PSC is more common than was previously believed. However, there are no clear indications of a true increase in the prevalence of PSC among patients with UC[6]. An association with Crohn's disease was suggested by Atkinson and Carroll as early as 1964; this association has been less well recognized[7]. Crohn's disease isolated to the small bowel (without colonic involvement) has, to the best of this author's knowledge, not been reported to be associated with PSC. In recent studies, 1.3–13% of patients with Crohn's disease have PSC[8–11]. It was suggested in a study from Norway that PSC may be seen as commonly in colonic Crohn's disease as in UC[12]. IBD can be diagnosed at any time during the course of PSC, and PSC can occur at any time during the course of IBD[13,14]. In general, however, IBD is diagnosed several years earlier than PSC. PSC may also develop many years after proctocolectomy in colitis and IBD can develop many years after liver transplantation[8,11,12,14,15]. There seems to be no correlation between the severity of UC and that of PSC[8,14].

In several studies, the prognostic significance of clinical, laboratory and histological parameters measured early in the course of PSC have been assessed using multivariate analysis[16–21]. Only in one of these studies has the presence of IBD been found to influence survival in patients with PSC[21]. It is of importance to point out that the patients included in the study by Wiesner and coworkers were later entered in a multicentre study evaluating the same prognostic variables; however, in this larger study, the presence of IBD did not have any influence on the outcome in PSC patients with IBD[17]. Thus, associated IBD in patients with PSC does not seem to influence survival.

PREVALENCE OF IBD IN PATIENTS WITH PSC

There is a wide global range of the prevalence of UC in patients with PSC, varying from 21–23% (reported from Japan)[22,23], 44% (in Spain)[24], 50% (in India)[25] 71% (in US)[21], to as much as 98% (in Norway)[19] (Table 1). The prevalence of PSC in patients with IBD and persistent abnormal liver function tests also varies (between 2.4% and 7.5%)[10,12,26,27]. Thus, the prevalence of IBD in PSC and the prevalence of PSC in IBD varies greatly between different studies. When comparing the different studies, one has to keep in mind that PSC can be present as an asymptomatic disease with only a mild deterioration of liver function, and that the abnormalities may fluctuate, so that episodes of normal liver function may occur. Therefore, the prevalence of PSC in patients with IBD will depend on the number of patients being screened by liver function tests and how frequently these tests are made[6]. Causes other than PSC, such as autoimmune hepatitis and fatty change, may be present in IBC patients[28]. Furthermore, evidence of impaired liver function may be seen during colonic disease activity, treatment with steroids and total parenteral nutrition[6]. Therefore, registration with only liver function tests is not enough to estimate the prevalence of PSC in patients with IBD; ideally, the tests should be made during an inactive stage of the colitis. When studying the prevalence of IBD in patients with PSC, it is important to note that the colitis in PSC patients is usually quiescent or mild[29]. All patients must undergo colonoscopic investigation in order to estimate the prevalence of IBD in PSC. In studies from Norway in which all patients have been investigated with colonoscopy, 98% of the patients with PSC were found to have colitis. However,

Table 1 Frequency of IBD in patients with PSC in different parts of the world

First author	*Country*	*Number of patients*	*IBD (%)*	*UC (%)*	*Crohn's (%)*	*Unclassified colitis (%)*
Schrumpf[19]	Norway	77	98	75	14	9
Broomé[16]	Sweden	305	81	72	7	2
Farrant[18]	England	126	73	71	2	–
Wiesner[11]	USA	174	71	–	–	–
Okolicsanyi[55]	Italy	117	54	36	10	8
Kochar[25]	India	18	50	–	–	–
Escorsell[24]	Spain	43	46	44	2	–
Takikawa[23]	Japan	192	21	20	1	–

in a study from the US, also in which all patients had been investigated with colonoscopy, only 71% of them had colitis[12,30]. Differences may exist in the association between IBD and PSC in different parts of the world.

COMPARISONS BETWEEN PSC PATIENTS WITH AND WITHOUT IBD

In a study of liver biopsies and autopsy specimens from 43 PSC patients with and without UC, and 19 UC patients with abnormal liver function tests but normal cholangiograms, Ludwig *et al.* found essentially the same morphological features whether PSC was or was not associated with UC[31]. The authors therefore suggested that the causes of these conditions are closely related. MacCarty *et al.* could not find any differences in the radiological features of PSC patients with and without IBD[32]. However, Rabinovitz and coworkers, who investigated patients mostly with advanced PSC, found that there were significant differences between PSC patients with and without IBD[30]. Patients with PSC associated with IBD were more likely to be male and to present with abnormal liver function as the first manifestation of the liver disease, whereas jaundice, pruritus and fatigue were the primary symptoms in those patients without IBD. This finding may well reflect the fact that most UC patients today are regularly screened with liver function tests and PSC in patients with IBD is therefore diagnosed before the onset of liver-related symptoms. Furthermore, Rabinovitz *et al.* showed that the location of the bile-duct involvement in PSC differed significantly between the two groups. Combined intrahepatic and extrahepatic bile duct strictures were found more frequently in patients with IBD than in those without IBD (82% vs. 46%). In contrast, involvement of the extrahepatic bile ducts alone was more frequent in patients without IBD (38% vs. 7%). Still, these findings do not seem to be sufficient to conclude that PSC, occurring in patients without IBD, is an entity separate from PSC found in association with IBD.

COMPARISONS OF UC IN PATIENTS WITH AND WITHOUT PSC

The prevalence of PSC is 5.5% in patients with substantial colitis and 0.5% in patients with distal colitis[26]. Moreover, 95% of all PSC patients with UC have substantial colitis and only 5% have distal involvement, which differs significantly from UC patients without PSC[26].

In a case–control study, 29 PSC patients with extensive colitis were each matched with two UC patients without liver disease in order to compare the course of colitis in UC patients with and without PSC. The patients were followed regularly for approximately 20 years and it was found that UC in patients with PSC generally runs a quiescent course compared with UC patients without PSC[29]. In another Swedish study including 76 PSC patients, 52 were found to have UC, 8 Crohn's disease, and 11 patients did not have any clinical signs or history of IBD[13]. Nine of these asymptomatic patients underwent colonoscopy with multiple biopsies. Seven patients had endoscopic and/or histological signs of IBD. Among them, one had dysplasia and another epithelial changes probably positive for dysplasia. During follow-up, 2 patients died before development of bowel symptoms but 3 patients developed clinical symptoms of IBD 1–7 years after the first colonoscopy. Thus, the onset of IBD may have a substantial subclinical phase, leading to underestimation of disease duration and delay in inclusion of PSC patients with extensive colitis into surveillance programmes unless all PSC patients undergo colonoscopic investigation with multiple biopsies. Moreover, the subclinical phase may allow the study of early pathogenesis of IBD *in vivo*. Colonoscopic investigation is further warranted since a normal outcome in investigations with barium enema is seen in a high proportion of patients with PSC and IBD[8]. Furthermore, proctosigmoidoscopy as the sole means of investigation is insufficient in diagnosing UC in patients with PSC, since one study found that, in 23% of the PSC + UC patients, the rectum was spared[33].

COLECTOMY IN PATIENTS WITH IBD AND PSC

The effect of proctocolectomy on disease progression in patients with UC and PSC was addressed in a study by Cangemi *et al.*[34]. Clinical, histological, biochemical and cholangiographic features were compared between 20 PSC patients with UC who had undergone proctocolectomy and 25 PSC patients with UC but no proctocolectomy. It was found that proctocolectomy for UC appears to have little or no effect on the progression of PSC. Martin *et al.* came to the same conclusion since no difference in survival was found between 39 PSC patients who had undergone colectomy compared with 49 unoperated patients[35]. However, in a study from Finland, the liver involvement and its course after proctocolectomy were investigated in 13 patients with PSC and 14 patients with mild or moderate cholangitis or periportal hepatitis[36]. In repeated liver biopsies after proctocolectomy, active inflammation disappeared in some cases, especially when the primary findings were mild. More advanced findings, both on histology and cholangiography, remained unchanged or progressed with time.

A special complication of portal hypertension in PSC patients with a history of colectomy with an ileal stoma is the development of peristomal varices. The majority of the patients developing peristomal varices also suffer from oesophageal varices[37,38]. The peristomal varices develop within the adhesions between the ileal (portal) veins and the anterior abdominal wall (systemic) veins[39]. The bleeding occurs from the peristomal mucocutaneous junction. Patients bleeding from peristomal varices often present with recurrent haemorrhagic episodes, bleeding from the peristomal varices being more difficult to treat successfully than oesophageal varices. Local treatments to control bleeding are usually unsuccessful in the long run[38]. Peristomal variceal bleeding can be controlled with a portosystemic shunt, but if a PSC patient presents with peristomal varices, the severity of the liver disease is an indication for liver transplantation as the most appropriate treatment. It has been suggested that ileostomy should be avoided in PSC patients requiring proctocolectomy and that ileoanal, ileorectal or ileal pouch–anal anastomosis, which are less susceptible to variceal formation and bleeding, are to be preferred in these patients[40]. Nonspecific inflammation of the pouch (pouchitis) is the most frequent long-term complication in UC patients operated on with an ileal pouch–anal anastomosis. Patients with PSC are more likely to have chronic pouchitis (60%) than UC patients without PSC (15%)[41]. The risk of pouchitis is not related to the severity of the liver disease. Patients with small bile duct PSC develop pouchitis less often than those with large duct PSC[41]. In PSC patients having pouchitis before liver transplantation, most continue to have pouchitis after transplantation in spite of triple immunosuppression treatment, suggesting that antibiotic, rather than immune-modifying therapy, is the treatment of choice for pouchitis[42]. The association between PSC and pouchitis may suggest that a common pathogenetic mechanism is involved in both conditions.

COLORECTAL DYSPLASIA/CARCINOMA IN PATIENTS WITH UC AND PSC

It is well known that patients with UC have an increased risk of developing colorectal carcinoma. The two major risk factors for this complication are long duration of disease and extensive colitis. The cause of neoplastic change in UC remains unexplained. Lately, the presence of PSC has been shown to increase the risk of colorectal cancer/dysplasia in patients with UC[43–47]. In a study from Sweden, the absolute cumulative risk of developing colorectal dysplasia/cancer in the PSC/UC group was 9%, 31% and 50%, respectively, after 10, 20 and 25 years of disease duration. In the group with UC only, the corresponding risk was 2%, 5% and 10%, respectively[44]. Almost identical cumulative incidence of colorectal neoplasia was found in a recent Finnish case–control study, including 45 patients with UC and concomitant PSC and 45 pair-matched control patients with UC only[47]. The cumulative incidence of colorectal neoplasia was 11% at 10 years and 31% at 20 years from onset of disease in the group with UC and PSC, and 3% at 10 years and 8% at 20 years in the control group of UC patients without PSC ($p<0.01$). However, contradictory results have also been presented from the Mayo Clinic[48]. One hundred and seventy eight patients with PSC were identified and stratified by geographical area of residence and were followed up to determine development of colorectal carcinoma. Comparisons were made with a previous study in which the risk of colorectal cancer in UC has been assessed in a large cohort of UC patients (also including patients with PSC)[49]. Among the 178 PSC patients, no increased risk for the development of colorectal carcinoma was found compared with UC patients. However, among the 178 PSC patients, only 143 patients had UC. In the subgroup of PSC patients with UC, the cumulative incidence of colorectal carcinoma and dysplasia was 20% at 20 years and 67% at 30 years after diagnosis of UC, indicating that also in this study PSC patients with UC have an increased risk of developing colorectal neoplasia. PSC patients with UC remain at an increased risk of developing colon cancer/dysplasia even after they have undergone liver transplantation[50,51].

Cholangiocarcinoma, the most feared long-term complication in PSC, was found in one study to develop more often in PSC patients with colonic dysplasia/carcinoma[44]. This finding may suggest that patients with PSC and UC with colonic dysplasia/carcinoma may constitute a high-risk subgroup for development of cholangiocarcinoma. If this is confirmed by further studies, the finding of colonic dysplasia in patients with PSC and UC may reduce the threshold for referring PSC patients for liver transplantation.

It is of importance to emphasize the necessity that all patients with PSC and UC be included in colonoscopic surveillance programmes, probably at an earlier time than UC patients without PSC. Also, after transplantation, an annual colonoscopy of these patients is recommended.

INFLAMMATORY BOWEL DISEASE AND PSC IN PATIENTS UNDERGOING LIVER TRANSPLANTATION

In studies investigating the relationship between PSC and UC after liver transplantation, conflicting data have been found. In one study from Los Angeles including 29 PSC patients with UC who were liver transplanted, it was found that the course of the colonic disease was not altered after transplantation[52]. Moreover, active ulcerative colitis did not adversely affect allograft function although alkaline phosphatase increased significantly in UC patients with active UC compared with those with inactive disease[52]. In another American study including 23 PSC patients with UC who were liver transplanted, it was shown that symptoms of UC severity significantly improved following liver transplantation with immunosuppression with cyclosporin and prednisone[53].

The question of whether the presence of IBD affects the outcome after liver transplantation in patients with PSC was addressed in a study from Birmingham[54]. Among 55 PSC patients undergoing liver transplantation, 31 of the patients had associated IBD[54]. After liver transplantation, there were significantly more episodes of acute rejection in the patients with IBD than in those without IBD. The number of patients with chronic rejection did not differ between PSC patients with and without IBD. The frequency of recurrent PSC after liver transplantation and 5-year survival did not differ between PSC patients with and without associated IBD.

CONCLUSIONS

The prevalence of IBD in patients with PSC differs considerably in various parts of the world. Ulcerative colitis is seen most frequently but 1–14% of all PSC patients have Crohn's disease with colonic involvement. The characteristics of IBD in patients with PSC differ concerning several factors: the colitis is usually substantial, and the clinical course of the colitis is quiescent. Many PSC patients without clinical symptoms of IBD have colonoscopic and histological findings compatible with IBD and the subclinical phase may last up to seven years before the onset of symptoms of active colitis. PSC patients with UC have an increased risk of developing colorectal dysplasia/carcinoma compared with UC patients without PSC. Moreover, PSC patients undergoing ileal-J anal anastomosis have a significantly increased risk of developing pouchitis. It is of importance that all PSC patients with UC are included in colonoscopic surveillance programmes.

References

1. Thomas C. Ulceration of the colon with a much enlarged fatty liver. Trans Pathol Soc Philadelphia. 1873;4:87–8.
2. Ross J, Swarts J. Hepatic dysfunction and cirrhosis in chronic ulcerative colitis. Gastroenterology. 1948;10:81–95.
3. Kimmelstein P, Large H. Liver damage in ulcerative colitis. Am J Pathol. 1952;28:259–74.
4. Smith M, Loe R. Sclerosing cholangitis. Am J Surg. 1965;110:239–46.
5. Warren K, Athanassiades S, Monge J. Primary sclerosing cholangitis. A study of forty-two cases. Am J Surg. 1966;111:23–38.
6. Broomé U, Glaumann H, Hellers G, Nilsson B, Sörstad J, Hultcrantz R. Liver disease in ulcerative colitis: an epidemiological and follow-up study in the county of Stockholm. Gut. 1994;35: 84–9.
7. Atkinson A, Carroll W. Sclerosing cholangitis associated with regional enteritis. JAMA. 1964; 188:183–4.
8. Chapman RWG, Arborgh BAM, Rhodes JM *et al.* Primary sclerosing cholangitis; a review of its clinical features, cholangiography and hepatic histology. Gut. 1980;21:870–7.
9. Rasmussen H, Fallingberg J, Mortensen P, Vyberg M, Tage-Jenssen U, Rasmussen S. Hepatobiliary dysfunction and presence of primary sclerosing cholangitis in patients with Crohn's disease. Scand J Gastroenterol. 1997;32:604–10.
10. Tobias R, Wright J, Kottler R. Primary sclerosing cholangitis associated with inflammatory bowel disease in Cape Town, 1975–1981. S Afr Med J. 1983;63:229–35.
11. Wiesner RH, LaRusso NF. Clinicopathologic features of the syndrome of primary sclerosing cholangitis. Gastroenterology. 1980;1980:200–6.
12. Aadland E, Schrumpf E, Fausa O *et al.* Primary sclerosing cholangitis: a long-term follow-up study. Scand J Gastroenterol. 1987;22:655–64.
13. Broomé U, Löfberg R, Lundqvist K, Veress B. Subclinical time span of inflammatory bowel disease in patients with primary sclerosing cholangitis. Dis Colon Rectum. 1995;38:1301–5.
14. Fausa O, Schrumpf E, Elgjo K. Relationship of inflammatory bowel disease and primary sclerosing cholangitis. Semin Liver Dis. 1991;11:31–9.
15. Wiesner R, Porayko M, Hay J *et al.* Liver transplantation for primary sclerosing cholangitis: impact of risk factors on outcome. Liver Transplant Surg. 1996;2:99–108.
16. Broomé U, Olsson R, Lööf L *et al.* Natural history and prognostic factors in 305 Swedish patients with primary sclerosing cholangitis. Gut. 1996;38:610–15.
17. Dickson ER, Murtaugh PA, Wiesner RH *et al.* Primary sclerosing cholangitis: refinement and validation of survival models. Gastroenterology. 1992;103:1893–901.
18. Farrant JM, Hayllar KM Wilkinson ML *et al.* Natural history and prognostic variables in primary sclerosing cholangitis. Gastroenterology. 1991;100:1710–17.
19. Schrumpf E, Abdelnoor M, Fausa O, Elgjo K, Jenssen E, Kolmannskog F. Risk factors in primary sclerosing cholangitis. J Hepatol. 1994;21:1061–6.
20. Shetty K, Rybicki L, Carey W. The Child–Pugh classification as a prognostic indicator for survival in primary sclerosing cholangitis. Hepatology. 1997;25:1049–53.
21. Wiesner RH, Grambsch PM, Dickson R *et al.* Primary sclerosing cholangitis: natural history, prognostic factors and survival analysis. Hepatology. 1989;10:430–6.
22. Okada H, Mizuno M, Yamamoto K, Tsuji T. Primary sclerosing cholangitis in Japanese patients: Association with inflammatory bowel disease. Acta Med Oktayama. 1996;50:227–35.
23. Takikawa H, Manabe T. Primary sclerosing cholangitis in Japan – analysis of 192 cases. J Gastroenterol. 1997;32:134–7.
24. Escorsell A, Pares A, Rodes J, Soli-Herruzo J, Miras M, de la Morena E. Epidemiology of primary sclerosing cholangitis in Spain. J Hepatol. 1994;21:787–91.
25. Kochhar R, Goenka M, Das K *et al.* Primary sclerosing cholangitis: an experience from India. J Gastroenterol Hepatol. 1996;11:429–33.
26. Olsson R, Danielsson A, Jarnerot G *et al.* Prevalence of primary sclerosing cholangitis in patients with ulcerative colitis. Gastroenterology. 1991;100:1319–23.
27. Shepherd H, Selby W, Chapman R *et al.* Ulcerative colitis and persistent liver dysfunction. Q J Med. 1983;52:503–13.
28. Schrumpf E, Fausa O, Elgjo K, Kolmannskog F. Hepatobiliary complications of inflammatory bowel disease. Semin Liver Dis. 1988;8:201–9.

29. Lundqvist K, Broomé U. Differences in colonic disease activity in patients with ulcerative colitis with and without primary sclerosing cholangitis. Dis Colon Rectum. 1997;40:451–6.
30. Rabinovitz M, Gavaler JS, Schade RR, Dindzans VJ, Chien MC, Van Thiel DH. Does primary sclerosing cholangitis occurring in association with inflammatory bowel disease differ from that occurring in the absence of inflammatory bowel disease? A study of sixty-six subjects. Hepatology. 1990;11:7–11.
31. Ludwig J, Barham SS, La Russo NF, Elveback LR, Wiesner RH, McCall JT. Morphologic features of chronic hepatitis associated with primary sclerosing cholangitis and chronic ulcerative colitis. Hepatology. 1981;1:632–40.
32. MacCarty R, LaRusso N, Wiesner R, Ludwig J. Primary sclerosing cholangitis: findings on cholangiography and pancreatography. Radiology. 1983;149:39–44.
33. Perdigoto R, Wiesner R, LaRusso N, Dozois R. Inflammatory bowel disease associated with primary sclerosing cholangitis: incidence, severity and relationship to liver disease (abstr). Gastroenterology. 1991;100:A238.
34. Cangemi J, Wiesner R, Beaver S *et al.* Effect of proctocolectomy for chronic ulcerative colitis on the natural history of primary sclerosing cholangitis. Gastroenterology. 1989;96:790–4.
35. Martin FM, Rossi RL, Nugent FW *et al.* Surgical aspects of sclerosing cholangitis. Results in 178 patients. Ann Surg. 1990;212:551–6.
36. Mikkola K, Kiviluoto T, Riihela M, Taavitsainen M, Jarvinen HJ. Liver involvement and its course in patients operated on for ulcerative colitis. Hepatogastroenterology. 1995;42:68–72.
37. Fucini C, Wolff B, Dozois R. Bleeding from peristomal varices: perspectives on prevention and treatment. Dis Colon Rectum. 1991;34:1073–8.
38. Wiesner RH, La Russo NF, Dozois RR, Beaver SJ. Peristomal varices after proctocolectomy in patients with primary sclerosing cholangitis. Gastroenterology. 1986;90:316–22.
39. Peck JJ, Boyden AM. Exigent ileostomy hemorrhage. A complication of proctocolectomy in patients with chronic ulcerative colitis and primary sclerosing cholangitis. Am J Surg. 1985; 150:153–8.
40. Kartheuser AH, Dozois RR, La Russo NF, Wiesner RH, Ilstrup DM, Schleck CD. Comparison of surgical treatment of ulcerative colitis associated with primary sclerosing cholangitis: ileal pouch–anal anastomosis versus Brooke ileostomy. Mayo Clin Proc. 1996;71:748–56.
41. Penna C, Dozios R, Tremaine W *et al.* Pouchitis after ileal pouch–anal anastomosis for ulcerative colitis occurs with increased frequency in patients with associated primary sclerosing cholangitis. Gut. 1996;38:234–9.
42. Zins BJ, Sandborn WJ, Penna CR *et al.* Pouchitis disease course after orthotopic liver transplantation in patients with primary sclerosing cholangitis and an ileal pouch–anal anastomosis. Am J Gastroenterol. 1995;90:2177–81.
43. Broomé U, Lindberg G, Löfberg R. Primary sclerosing cholangitis in ulcerative colitis – a risk factor for the development of dysplasia and DNA aneuploidy? Gastroenterology. 1992;102: 1877–80.
44. Broomé U, Löfberg R, Veress B, Eriksson LS. Primary sclerosing cholangitis and ulcerative colitis: evidence for increased neoplastic potential. Hepatology. 1995;22:1404–8.
45. Brentnall TA, Haggitt RC, Rabinovitch PS *et al.* Risk and natural history of colonic neoplasia in patients with primary sclerosing cholangitis and ulcerative colitis. Gastroenterology. 1996;110: 331–8.
46. D'Haens GR, Lashner BA, Hanauer SB. Pericholangitis and sclerosing cholangitis are risk factors for dysplasia and cancer in ulcerative colitis. Am J Gastroenterol. 1993;88:1174–8.
47. Leidenius M, Färkkilä M, Kärkkäinen P, Taskinen E, Kellokumpu I, Höckerstedt K. Colorectal dysplasia and carcinoma in patients with ulcerative colitis and primary sclerosing cholangitis. Scand J Gastroenterol. 1997;32:706–11.
48. Loftus EV Jr, Sandborn WJ, Tremaine WJ *et al.* Risk of colorectal neoplasia in patients with primary sclerosing cholangitis. Gastroenterology. 1996;110:432–40.
49. Ekbom A, Helmick C, Zack M, Adami H. Ulcerative colitis and colorectal cancer. N Engl J Med. 1990;323:1228–33.
50. Bleday R, Lee E, Jessurun J, Heine J, Wong WD. Increased risk of early colorectal neoplasms after hepatic transplant in patients with inflammatory bowel disease. Dis Colon Rectum. 1993; 36:908–12.
51. Higashi H, Yanaga K, Marsh JW, Tzakis A, Kakizoe S, Starzl TE. Development of colon cancer after liver transplantation for primary sclerosing cholangitis associated with ulcerative colitis.

Hepatology. 1990;11:477–80.

52. Shaked A, Colonna JO, Goldstein L, Busuttil RW. The interrelation between sclerosing cholangitis and ulcerative colitis in patients undergoing liver transplantation. Ann Surg. 1992; 215:598–603.
53. Gavaler JS, Delemos B, Belle SH *et al.* Ulcerative colitis disease activity as subjectively assessed by patient-completed questionnaires following orthotopic liver transplantation for sclerosing cholangitis. Dig Dis Sci. 1991;36:321–8.
54. Miki C, Harrison JD, Gunson BK, Buckels JA, McMaster P, Mayer AD. Inflammatory bowel disease in primary sclerosing cholangitis: an analysis of patients undergoing liver transplantation. Br J Surg. 1995;82:1114–17.
55. Okolicsanyi L, Fabris L, Viaggi S *et al.* Primary sclerosing cholangitis: clinical presentation, natural history and prognostic variables. An Italian multicenter study. Eur J Gastroenterol Hepatol. 1996;8:685–91.

8
Risk of cholangiocarcinoma in primary sclerosing cholangitis

S. M. RIORDAN and R. WILLIAMS

INTRODUCTION

Primary sclerosing cholangitis (PSC) is a chronic liver disorder of unknown aetiology, characterized by progressive obliterative fibrosis, usually involving both intra- and extrahepatic bile ducts and occurring predominantly in young adults[1,2]. The natural history is variable, with some asymptomatic patients having disease which does not progress over extended periods of time. However, the serious and progressive nature of PSC in the majority of cases can be surmised from estimates of overall median survival, ranging from 12 to 21 years[3–6], depending on differences in definitions of starting points as well as in referral patterns and patient recruitment, which represent a reduced life expectancy of about 30 years[4]. Liver transplantation is an effective and commonly used treatment option for advanced disease, 21% of PSC patients in one series having undergone transplantation at a median of 6.5 years (range: 1–22 years) after first presentation[3], and PSC is now among the most common indications for liver transplantation in both the northern and southern hemispheres[3,7–10].

PSC is strongly associated with inflammatory bowel disease (IBD), predominantly ulcerative colitis, which is present in approximately 75% of PSC patients. Conversely, between 5% and 10% of patients with ulcerative colitis have or will develop PSC[2,11,12]. An association between IBD and cholangiocarcinoma has long been recognized, with cholangiocarcinoma reported in approximately 0.5% of patients with ulcerative colitis, in whom the relative risk of cholangiocarcinoma development has been estimated to be over 31 times that of the general population[13,14]. The finding of cholangiocarcinoma was previously considered by definition to preclude a diagnosis of PSC, but, with increasing knowledge of the natural history of PSC, there has developed a substantial body of evidence that, not only are patients with this disorder at increased risk of developing cholangiocarcinoma, but the increased risk of cholangiocarcinoma in the setting of IBD occurs as a consequence of coincident PSC[15–17]. However, establishing a clinical diagnosis of cholangiocarcinoma in patients with PSC may be difficult and estimates of the magnitude of this increased risk vary appreciably between series according to the mode of tumour detection employed. This chapter reviews the literature concerning the prevalence of cholangiocarcinoma in PSC and the difficulties associated both with identifying PSC patients with cholangiocarcinoma in clinical practice and predicting which PSC patients are at particular risk of developing this tumour.

PREVALENCE OF CHOLANGIOCARCINOMA IN PATIENTS WITH PSC

The prevalence of cholangiocarcinoma in patients with PSC has been estimated to range from 5% to 15%[18]. However, many studies investigating this issue do not indicate whether prevalence figures are based on clinical assessment alone or on additional data obtained at autopsy, or, more recently, either at laparotomy for liver transplantation or by histological examination of livers explanted from transplant recipients. This is an important consideration in view of increasing evidence that prevalence figures obtained solely from clinical studies may substantially underestimate the true prevalence of cholangiocarcinoma in the setting of PSC. Indeed, it has been a common occurrence for this tumour to be detected only at autopsy in patients with PSC. For example, one study from the Mayo Clinic prospectively followed 70 patients with PSC entered into a randomized trial of medical treatment with D-penicillamine for a mean of 30 months[19]. Fifteen patients died during this period and autopsies were performed in 12. Cholangiocarcinoma was found in 5 of the 12 autopsied patients, in none of whom the diagnosis had been established during life. This gave an overall prevalence of 5/70 (7%), with the zero clinical detection rate substantially less than the 42% prevalence found in autopsied patients. Similarly, an English follow-up study of 29 patients with PSC over a longer mean follow-up period of 7 years found cholangiocarcinomas had developed in 3 patients over this time[17]. Each of these tumours was detected only at autopsy, which had been performed in 11 patients. Again, the overall prevalence of 10.3% was appreciably less than the 3/11 (27.3%) obtained by considering autopsy data. Aadland *et al.*[4] also reported an overall prevalence of cholangiocarcinoma of 4/45 (8.9%) in Swedish patients with PSC. All cases were again detected at autopsy, which was performed in 12 cases, giving an autopsy prevalence of 33.3%. In an epidemiological study of the incidence of ulcerative colitis in the county of Stockholm between 1955 and 1979, Broome *et al.*[5] identified 1274 patients with ulcerative colitis. Almost all patients had been regularly screened with measurement of liver enzyme levels in peripheral blood for hepatobiliary disease and abnormalities were detected in 142/1274 (11.1%) patients. PSC was eventually diagnosed in 29 (2.3%) patients. Twelve of these 29 patients died during the study period, 4 from cholangiocarcinoma. This gave an overall prevalence of cholangiocarcinoma in PSC of 4/29 (13.8%) and a prevalence from autopsy data of 4/12 (33.3%) (Table 1).

Studies in which explanted livers of transplant recipients have been examined histologically for clinically unsuspected cholangiocarcinoma have similarly highlighted the difficulties associated with establishing a clinical diagnosis of this tumour in the setting of PSC (Table 2). Farrant *et al.*[3] followed 126 patients with PSC who had presented at King's College Hospital between 1972 and 1989

Table 1 The prevalence of cholangiocarcinoma in patients with PSC, assessed clinically and at autopsy

Authors	*Location*	*Overall reported prevalence of cholangiocarcinoma (%)*	*Rate of clinical detection of cholangiocarcinoma (%)*	*Rate of cholangiocarcinoma detection at autopsy (%)*
Rosen *et al.*[19]	USA	5/70 (7.1)	0/70 (0.0)	5/12 (41.7)
Chapman *et al.*[17]	England	3/29 (10.3)	0/29 (0.0)	3/11 (27.3)
Aadland *et al.*[4]	Sweden	4/45 (8.9)	0/45 (0.0)	4/12 (33.3)
Broome *et al.*[5]	Sweden	4/29 (13.8)	NS	4/12 (33.3)

NS: not stated

for a median period of 5.8 years. During this time, there were more patients who underwent liver transplantation (21%) than died of liver-related disease (16%). Overall, cholangiocarcinoma was found in 8/126 (6.3%) patients, including 6/26 (23.1%) patients who underwent transplantation. In only 2 of these latter patients had the cholangiocarcinoma been detected clinically, the other 4 cases being found only on subsequent histological examination of the explanted livers despite a rigorous pretransplant assessment. An additional 31 patients later underwent liver transplantation for PSC at the same centre between 1989 and 1994[20]. Although the number of patients with clinically occult cholangiocarcinoma, evident only on subsequent histological examination of the hepatectomy specimen, had fallen from 4/26 (15.4%) in the early series to 1/31 (3.2%), this difference was not statistically significant and the prevalence of cholangiocarcinomas detectable only in the explanted liver, rather than clinically, remained high, namely 50.0%.

This has also been a common experience in other series reported from other centres. Abu-Elmagd *et al.*[21] reported a large series of 169 consecutive patients with PSC who underwent liver transplantation at the University of Pittsburgh Medical Centre from 1981 to 1990. Eighteen of these patients (10.7%) were found to have a concomitant cholangiocarcinoma. The tumour was intrahepatic in 2 (11.1%) patients, hilar in 13 (72.2%) patients and involved gallbladder or cystic duct in 3 (16.6%) patients. However, the diagnosis of cholangiocarcinoma could be established preoperatively in only 7/169 (4.1%) patients. A thorough histological examination of the hepatectomy specimen revealed the clinically unsuspected coexistence of cholangiocarcinoma in an additional 11 (6.5%) patients, such that over 61% of cholangiocarcinomas in this series were not detected by clinical means alone.

In a study of 305 Swedish patients with PSC, all of whom were followed for a median time of 63 months, Broome *et al.*[22] reported a prevalence of cholangiocarcinoma in PSC of 12/34 (35.3%), as determined by histological examination of the explanted livers of transplant recipients. In addition, cholangiocarcinoma was the main cause of death in 12/45 (26.7%) patients who had died without undergoing liver transplantation during the follow-up period. Thus, among the 79 patients who died or underwent liver transplantation, cholangiocarcinoma had developed in 24 (30.4%).

Table 2 Prevalences of cholangiocarcinoma detected clinically and at laparotomy or in the explanted livers of patients with PSC undergoing orthotopic liver transplantation (OLT)

			Patients with			
Authors	*Location*	*No. undergoing OLT*	*Cholangiocarcinoma detected clinically prior to OLT (%)*	*Cholangiocarcinoma present at laparotomy or in explanted liver (%)*	*Clinically occult cholangiocarcinoma (%)*	*Cholangiocarcinomas not detected clinically (%)*
Farrant *et al.*[3]	England	26	2/26 (7.7)	6/26 (23.1)	4/26 (15.4)	4/6 (66.7)
Muiesan *et al.*[20]	England	31	1/31 (3.2)	2/31 (6.5)	1/31 (3.2)	½ (50.0)
Abu-Elmagd *et al.*[21]	USA	169	7/169 (4.1)	18/169 (10.7)	11/169 (6.5)	11/18 (61.1)
Broome *et al.*[22]	Sweden	34	NS	12/34 (35.3)	NS	NS
Miros *et al.*[10]	Australia	11	1/11 (9.1)	4/11 (36.4)	3/11 (27.3)	3/4 (75.0)
Marsh *et al.*[9]	USA	55	0/55 (0.0)	5/55 (9.1)	5/55 (9.1)	5/5 (100.0)
Knechtle *et al.*[23]	USA	41	2/41 (4.9)	6/41 (14.6)*	5/41 (12.2)	5/7 (71.4)
Broome and Eriksson[8]	Sweden	10	0/11 (0.0)	3/11 (27.3)	3/11 (27.3)	3/3 (100.0)
Ismail *et al.*[24]	England	17	0/17 (0.0)	2/17 (11.8)	2/17 (11.8)	2/2 (100.0)
Narumi *et al.*[25]	US	34	0/34 (0.0)	1/34 (2.9)	1/34 (2.9)	1/1 (100.0)

NS: not stated. *One of the two patients with cholangiocarcinoma detected clinically prior to OLT underwent treatment with radiotherapy and chemotherapy and no tumour was subsequently found in the explanted liver

Miros *et al.*[10] investigated the prevalence of cholangiocarcinoma in 11 PSC patients who underwent liver transplantation at an Australian centre between 1985 and 1989. Cholangiocarcinoma had been confirmed pretransplantation by fine-needle aspiration cytology in 1/11 (9.1%) patients. A second patient was found to have cholangiocarcinoma at the time of laparotomy for transplantation, and, in 2 additional patients in whom no evidence of tumour was found at laparotomy, the diagnosis was reached only by microscopic examination of the hepatectomy specimen. Thus, 3/11 (27.3%) patients had clinically occult cholangiocarcinoma, whilst 3/4 (75.0%) instances of cholangiocarcinoma were not detected clinically in this series. Tumours were located in the common hepatic duct with local invasion into both lobes of the liver in one patient, the common bile duct in one patient, common bile and hepatic ducts in one patient and common bile and hepatic ducts along with adjacent liver in the other patient. All patients had evidence of extensive intraneural and perineural spread, with microscopic involvement of the portal vein in two patients.

Marsh *et al.*[9] also found a high prevalence of clinically unsuspected cholangiocarcinoma complicating PSC in 55 patients who underwent liver transplantation for recurrent variceal haemorrhage ($n=15$; 27.2%), ascending cholangitis ($n=15$; 27.2%) and hepatic decompensation, including encephalopathy, coagulopathy, ascites, pruritus and/or varices ($n=25$; 45.5%) at the University of Colorado Health Science Centre (during 1980), the University Health Centre of Pittsburgh (from 1981 to 1986) and the Pittsburgh-affiliated Baylor University Medical Centre at Dallas (from 1985 to 1986). Whilst cholangiocarcinoma had been diagnosed in no transplanted patient preoperatively, 5/55 (9.1%) were subsequently found to have this tumour when the hepatectomy specimen was examined histologically. Thus, all 5 (100%) tumours had not been detected clinically in this series.

Knechtle *et al.*[23] have reported their experience with cholangiocarcinoma in the setting of PSC since the inception of the liver transplant programme at the University of Wisconsin. Up to 1995, 41 patients with PSC had undergone liver transplantation at this centre. Almost all patients underwent transplantation electively, with only 4 (9.8%) patients being United Network of Organ Sharing status 4, implying emergency need for transplantation. Only 2 (4.9%) patients with a known preoperative diagnosis of cholangiocarcinoma underwent liver transplantation, one of whom had undergone combined radiotherapy and chemotherapy and had no evidence of tumour in the explanted liver. The other patient without gross tumour evident clinically had positive biliary brushings on cytological evaluation. In keeping with other studies, an additional 5 (12.2%) patients thought to have no evidence of malignancy clinically at the time of transplantation were found to have developed a cholangiocarcinoma when the hepatectomy specimen was examined histologically. Thus, over 71% of cholangiocarcinomas found in patients with PSC in this transplant programme were not detectable clinically.

Between 1985 and 1991, 37 patients with PSC were referred to Huddinge Hospital in Sweden for assessment for liver transplantation[8]. Eleven patients without clinical evidence of cholangiocarcinoma underwent laparotomy with a view to proceeding to transplantation. Cholangiocarcinoma was found in 3/11 (27.3%) patients, one with evidence of extrahepatic spread at laparotomy, in whom transplantation was not proceeded with, and two with small intrahepatic cholangiocarcinomas evident only in the explanted liver.

Forty-eight patients with PSC were assessed at Queen Elizabeth Hospital in Birmingham between 1984 and 1989[24]. Liver transplantation was performed in 17 patients over this time. Although no transplanted patient was considered to have cholangiocarcinoma on clinical grounds during evaluation for transplantation, a tumour was subsequently detected in 2/17 (11.8%) patients, one of whom had evidence of metastatic disease at laparotomy and the other in whom the cholangiocarcinoma became evident only when the explanted liver was examined histologically.

The lowest percentage of PSC patients with clinically occult cholangiocarcinomas found only at laparotomy for liver transplantation or in the explanted liver has been reported by Narumi *et al.* at the University of California[25]. Thirty-four patients in whom cholangiocarcinoma had not been documented clinically underwent laparotomy between 1988 and 1993 with a view to proceeding to liver transplantation. PSC had been diagnosed a median of 60 months (range: 2–262 months) prior to surgery. The transplant procedure was abandoned in one patient with obvious tumour mass with metastatic spread at laparotomy. However, no additional cholangiocarcinomas were identified despite careful histological evaluation of the hepatectomy specimens, which included as much host common bile duct and surrounding nodal tissue as possible. It is not stated whether the preoperative investigative regimen or patient selection criteria employed in this study differed in any way from those used in some of the other studies discussed above, in which substantially higher prevalences of 'incidental' cholangiocarcinomas in hepatic explants were reported.

DIFFICULTIES IN THE CLINICAL DETECTION OF CHOLANGIOCARCINOMA

The discrepancies highlighted above demonstrate the inadequacies of currently employed modalities for the clinical detection of cholangiocarcinoma in patients with PSC. This is due, at least in part, to the fact that signs and symptoms of cholangiocarcinoma complicating PSC are non-specific. In particular, the most common symptoms and signs in patients with PSC complicated by cholangiocarcinoma are similar to those present in patients with PSC alone[17,19] (Tables 3 and 4). The only symptom identified by Broome *et al.*[22] which occurred significantly more often in patients with cholangiocarcinoma than in the tumour-free group was abdominal pain, although this parameter was of little discriminant value in individual patients as it was present in only 59% of patients with cholangiocarcinoma and in 35% of those without a documented tumour.

Neither is there convincing evidence that any biochemical parameters reliably identify those PSC patients who had developed cholangiocarcinoma. The Queensland Transplant group reported that a rapid increase in levels of bilirubin and alkaline phosphatase are suggestive of the development of cholangiocarcinoma, although sample sizes were small and differences in levels of these parameters in PSC patients with and without superimposed cholangiocarcinoma did not reach statistical significance[10]. A larger Swedish study reported

Table 3 The most common symptoms in all patients with PSC and in those with PSC and confirmed cholangiocarcinoma

Symptom	*All patients with PSC (%)*[a]	*Patients with PSC and cholangiocarcinoma (%)*[b]
Jaundice	78	72
Weight loss	70	79
Abdominal pain	61	72
Pruritus	52	69

[a]From Chapman *et al.*[17]; [b]from Rosen *et al.*[19]

Table 4 Clinical signs in all patients with PSC assessed for liver transplantation and in the subgroup with PSC and confirmed cholangiocarcinoma[a]

Clinical sign	*All patients with PSC (%)*	*Patients with PSC and cholangiocarcinoma (%)*
Jaundice	65	78
Fever	27	33
Ascites	46	33
Hepatomegaly	57	78
Splenomegaly	24	22

[a]From Broome and Eriksson[8]

subsequently could not identify any biochemical parameters distinguishing PSC patients with cholangiocarcinoma from the group at large[8] (Table 5). Similarly, the Mayo Clinic series reported by Rosen *et al.*[19] could not identify any laboratory features which reliably indicated the presence of cholangiocarcinoma in individual patients with PSC. During the interval between the diagnoses of PSC and cholangiocarcinoma, progressive jaundice and at least a two-fold increase in alkaline phosphatase levels in peripheral blood occurred in 70% of patients, in keeping with the deterioration of otherwise stable disease noted in 73% of PSC patients with cholangiocarcinoma reported by Martin *et al.*[26]. However, up to 30% of PSC patients in these two series showed no change in any biochemical parameters with the appearance of the cholangiocarcinoma. Furthermore, the large Pittsburgh series reported by Abu-Elmagd *et al.*[21] could not retrospectively identify any laboratory differences in PSC patients undergoing liver transplantation who were subsequently found to have or not have cholangiocarcinomas in their explanted livers. There is also some suggestion that the increasing use of ursodeoxycholic acid in the treatment of PSC, which on present data improves the results of biochemical tests without otherwise influencing the natural history of PSC[27], may further complicate matters. Martins *et al.*[7] have reported 2 PSC patients on ursodeoxycholic acid who developed cholangiocarcinoma without the onset of jaundice or increase in peripheral blood levels of alkaline phosphatase or any other biochemical parameters. The initial suspicion of malignancy was based on the development of superficial thrombophlebitis and whether ursodeoxycholic acid may have masked any biochemical signs compatible with the development of cholangiocarcinoma, such as elevation of serum bilirubin or alkaline phosphatase levels, is speculative.

Table 5 Laboratory data in all patients with PSC assessed for liver transplantation and in the subgroup with PSC and confirmed cholangiocarcinoma[a]

Parameter	*Normal range*	*All patients with PSC* Mean (SEM)	*Patients with PSC and cholangiocarcinoma* Mean (SEM)[b]
Albumin (g/L)	35–46	24.9 (1.0)	25.4 (2.0)
Alkaline phosphatase (μmol/L)	<4.2	26.3 (3.4)	32.8 (9.2)
Bilirubin (μmol/L)	<26	208 (27)	203 (59)
Haemoglobin (g/dl)	13.0–16.5	11.3 (0.3)	11.6 (0.6)
Creatinine (μmol/L)	<120	105 (25)	85 (10)
Prothrombin index (%)	>130	79 (9)	78 (9)

[a]From Broome and Eriksson[8].
[b]No values in those with PSC and cholangiocarcinoma differed significantly from corresponding levels in the overall group

The ability of imaging techniques, including ultrasonography, computerized tomography and cholangiography, to detect cholangiocarcinoma in the setting of pre-existing PSC is also limited, although MacCarty *et al.*[28] reported one series from the Mayo Clinic in which marked bile duct dilatation was detected at cholangiography in all patients with cholangiocarcinoma complicating PSC. The presence of a polypoid mass at least 1 cm in diameter and progressive stricture formation or duct dilatation on serial cholangiograms were other findings which suggested the development of cholangiocarcinoma. Miros *et al.*[10] also found massive or progressive duct dilatation only in PSC patients with superimposed cholangiocarcinoma. However, others have not found these imaging criteria to be as reliable for identifying PSC patients with cholangiocarcinoma. Cholangiography was unable to detect cholangiocarcinoma in either of the 2 PSC patients with superimposed cholangiocarcinoma reported by Martins *et al.*[7], whilst Ramage *et al.*[29] detected only 4/15 (26.7%) cholangiocarcinomas in PSC patients using ultrasonography (sensitivity: 7%), computerized tomography (sensitivity: 29%) and endoscopic cholangiography (sensitivity: 58.3%). Further comparative studies are required to establish the value of magnetic resonance imaging[30]. The substantial prevalences of clinically occult cholangiocarcinomas in the liver transplantation and autopsy series discussed above, despite the use of imaging techniques, highlights the suboptimal sensitivity of cholangiography and other currently used imaging in this setting, probably because of the pre-existing distortion of the biliary tree. The difficulty in differentiating benign dominant biliary strictures from cholangiocarcinoma by cholangiographic appearance alone was demonstrated in one study of PSC patients awaiting liver transplantation, in whom ultrasound-guided biopsy of a dominant biliary stricture demonstrated benign disease in 25% of cases[31]. This observation is in keeping with reports by Miros *et al.*[10] and Ramage *et al.*[29], who found dominant biliary strictures in 43.0% and 42.8%, respectively, of patients subsequently transplanted for PSC, in whom superimposed cholangiocarcinoma was categorically excluded by histological examination of the explanted livers.

Cytological evaluations of aspirated bile or brushings of strictures at the time of endoscopic or percutaneous cholangiography have high specificities and positive predictive values for the diagnosis of cholangiocarcinoma in the non-PSC setting. However, low sensitivities and negative predictive values have been reported, such that negative results do not exclude the possibility of cholangiocarcinoma[32]. Comparative studies of bile and brush cytology performed in the non-PSC setting have reported sensitivities for cholangiocarcinoma of 11–30% and 50–56%, respectively[33,34]. The diagnostic accuracy was increased when samples were obtained on multiple occasions[35]. Cytological analysis of fine-needle aspirates obtained from strictured areas under imaging guidance yielded a sensitivity of 67%[33]. Mansfield *et al.* have more recently reported a sensitivity of 75% when multiple samples, including bile, biliary stricture brushings and secretions and washings from the proximal end of blocked biliary stents and the screw threads of stent retrievers, are examined in combination[36]. False-negative cytological results probably occur as a consequence of the scirrhous nature of cholangiocarcinoma, its tendency for submucosal spread and its often high degree of differentiation[37]. Few cytological studies have been performed in the PSC setting, although PSC was present in 22/65 (33.8%) patients with biliary strictures studied with brush cytology by Rabinovitz *et al.*[35]. Epithelial atypia due to PSC alone was reported and must be considered when interpreting results. The specificity, positive predictive value and overall accuracy of cytology for diagnosing cholangiocarcinoma in this specific circumstance remains to be determined.

In view of the difficulties in establishing the diagnosis of cholangiocarcinoma clinically by other means, several studies have been performed to investigate the value of measuring the tumour markers, carbohydrate antigen (CA) 19-9 and carcinoembryonic antigen (CEA) in the detection of cholangiocarcinoma. Nakeeb *et al.*[38] studied biliary CEA levels in, among others, 6 patients with PSC and 25 patients with confirmed cholangiocarcinoma (Table 6). Levels were significantly higher in patients with documented tumour (Figure 1). Biliary CEA levels were, apparently, not merely a reflection of the level of obstructive jaundice, as no significant correlation with serum levels of either bilirubin or alkaline phosphatase were found, although some concern as to the relevance of these findings was expressed in that several CEA-related glycoproteins present in normal human bile may have crossreacted with the CEA assay employed.

Nichols *et al.*[39] found serum CA 19-9 levels above 100 U/ml in 8/9 (88.9%) patients with PSC and superimposed cholangiocarcinoma (confirmed by fine-needle biopsy, $n=4$; at liver transplantation, $n=2$; at autopsy, $n=2$; and by brush cytology, $n=1$) compared with 4/28 (14.3%) patients with PSC alone, who were subsequently followed for a mean of 17.8 months. The sensitivity of a serum CA 19-9 level in excess of 100 U/ml for cholangiocarcinoma in PSC was 88.9%, whilst specificity was considered 85.7%, although longer follow-up times may have been required to definitively classify some patients as having 'false' positive levels. These authors considered measurement of serum CA 19-9 levels to be a promising test for the detection of cholangiocarcinoma. Of note, 2 patients in this series exhibited increased serum CA 19-9 levels approximately 6 months before the diagnosis of cholangiocarcinoma. These observations suggest that the tumour marker may have the potential to detect disease which is clinically occult by other methods.

Ramage *et al.*[29] subsequently reported the value of a combined index derived from serum levels of CA 19-9 and CEA for identifying patients with

Table 6 Clinical characteristics in patients in whom biliary carcinoembryonic antigen (CEA) levels were measured[a,b]

Biliary pathology	*n*	*Age* (years)	*Bilirubin* (mg/dl)	*ALP* (IU/ml)	*AST* (IU/ml)	*ALT* (IU/ml)
Benign structure	34	49±3.6	1.6±0.4	313±105	48±11	94±36
Choledochal cyst	5	31±6.0	0.4±0.1	117±19	36±16	41±8
Sclerosing cholangitis	6	56±5.4	2.5±1.0	356±137	66±23	76±26
Intrahepatic stones	5	60±7.7	2.4±1.2	488±311	44±13	70±38
Cholangiocarcinoma	25	68±2.4	6.8±1.5	403±63	117±36	101±21

Values expressed as mean±SEM. [a]From Nakeeb *et al.*[38]. [b]No significant differences in any values in patients with sclerosing cholangitis and cholangiocarcinoma

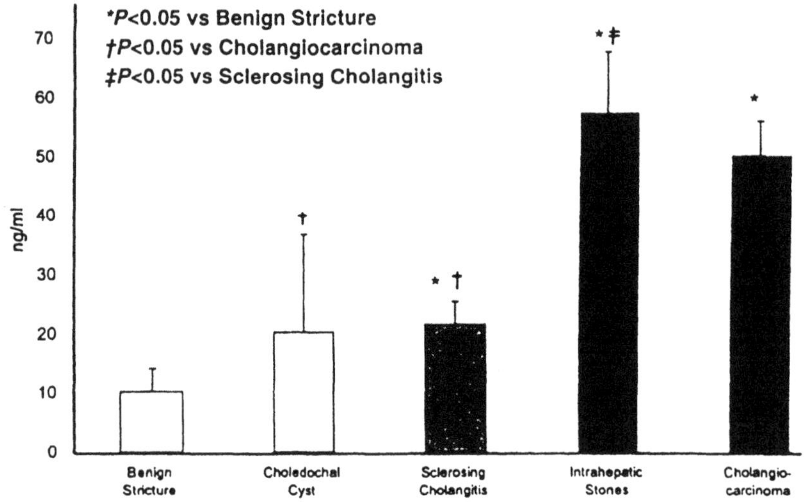

Figure 1 Mean hepatic bile carcinoembryonic antigen (CEA) concentrations in various patient groups. Levels in patients with PSC were significantly lower than those found in patients with confirmed cholangiocarcinoma[38]

cholangiocarcinoma. Three groups of patients were studied (Table 7). Group A consisted of 15 patients with histologically proven cholangiocarcinoma. Cholangiocarcinoma was diagnosed by imaging and biopsy in 4 (26.7%) patients, whilst tumours in the other 11 (73.3%) patients were not evident clinically or by ultrasonography, computerized tomography or endoscopic cholangiography at the time of presentation. Cholangiocarcinoma was diagnosed by histological examination of the explanted livers after transplantation in 8 of these patients, whilst tumour subsequently became evident after at least 3 months in the remaining 3 patients (either by imaging and biopsy or at postmortem examination). Group B comprised 22 patients with PSC severe enough to be treated by liver transplantation and who had no cholangiocarcinoma, as proven by histological examination of the explanted livers. This group was chosen for direct comparison with Group A as biochemical parameters were similar. Group

Table 7 Patient characteristics in three groups in whom a serum tumour marker index, based on CA 19-9 and CEA levels, was calculated[a]

	Group A Confirmed tumour	*Group B* Transplanted and no tumour	*Group C* Stable disease not requiring transplantation and no clinical evidence of tumour
n	15	22	37
Age (years)	42.5±8.1	41.2±9.9	43.9±15.4
Sex (M/F)	9/7	15/7	23/9
Bilirubin (μmol/L)	295.3±180.2	226.6±143.9	35.4±65.9
Albumin (g/L)	30.8±6.9	30.6±6.9	41.1±5.8
ALP (IU/L)	1200±559.9	785.4±488.6	456.4±429.6
Histological stage	3.1±1.1	3.8±0.4	2.6±1.0
Presence of inflammatory bowel disease (*n*)	8	11	24

Values expressed as mean±SD. [a]From Ramage *et al.*[29]

C consisted of 37 patients with stable PSC who had been followed for at least one year and in whom there was no clinical or radiological suspicion of cholangiocarcinoma. This group was studied in order to assess baseline values in PSC patients with stable disease. Using upper limit of normal values of 5 ng/ml for CEA and 200 U/ml for CA 19-9, the sensitivities of each marker for differentiating patients with superimposed cholangiocarcinoma (Group A) from those with no cholangiocarcinoma (Group B) was 53.3% for CEA and 60% for CA 19-9, with specificities of 86.3% and 91.0%, respectively. All patients with positive CEA values had colonic carcinoma excluded either by colonoscopy, barium enema or laparotomy.

An index combining these tumour markers was then derived using the formula CA 19-9+ (CEA×40), based on the best discriminant value for CA 19-9 (200 U/ml), which was 40 times that for CEA (5 ng/ml). The upper limit of normal for this index was arbitrarily chosen as 400. Values of the combined tumour marker index are shown in Figure 2. The ability of an index >400 to detect cholangiocarcinoma in PSC patients is shown in Table 8. Specificity and positive predictive value were each 100%. Sensitivity was only 66%, as values in patients with PSC and superimposed cholangiocarcinoma overlapped to some extent with those in patients with PSC alone. However, the high positive predictive value has clinical relevance in that a positive result suggests that cholangiocarcinoma is present. Furthermore, elevated values were found in 6/11 (54.5%) patients with clinically occult tumours (found only when the hepatectomy specimen was examined), suggesting that the majority of otherwise undiagnosed tumours can be detected by this index. The presumed diagnosis would have changed in 6/15 (40.0%) patients with cholangiocarcinoma if tumour markers had been tested at the time of presentation. It is unlikely that this index was elevated on the basis of increased CA 19-9 levels merely reflecting the degree of obstructive jaundice, as serum bilirubin levels were not significantly different in Group A and Group B patients and no significant correlation between serum bilirubin and CA 19-9 levels was found. Furthermore, immunohistochemical analysis has demonstrated

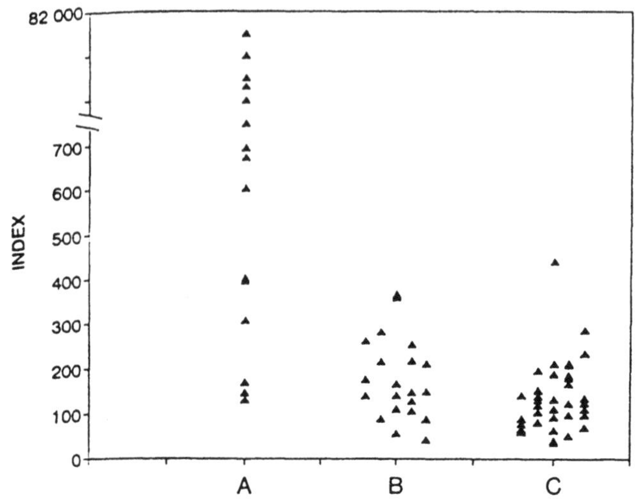

Figure 2 Values of the combined tumour marker index, based on consideration of serum CA 19-9 and CEA levels, in patients with primary sclerosing cholangitis (PSC) and confirmed cholangiocarcinoma (group A), those with severe PSC requiring transplantation but no cholangiocarcinoma (group B) and those with stable PSC not requiring liver transplantation (group C)[29]

Table 8 Reliability of the serum tumour marker index, based on CA 19-9 and CEA levels, for diagnosing cholangiocarcinoma in patients with PSC[a]

Tumour index	*Group A (confirmed cholangiocarcinoma)*	*Group B (no cholangiocarcinoma)*
>400	10	0
<400	5	22

Sensitivity:	66%
Specificity:	100%
Positive predictive value:	100%
Negative predictive value:	81%
Overall accuracy:	86%

[a]From Ramage *et al.*[29]

that 71% of cholangiocarcinomas stain positively for CA 19-9 and 91% for CEA, suggesting that the presence of an increased index based on these two tumour markers is due to the presence of tumour tissue rather than biliary obstruction.

Rizzi *et al.*[40] examined the expression of a mutant protein produced by the p53 tumour suppressor gene in PSC patients with and without superimposed cholangiocarcinoma. Using an immunohistochemical technique, expression of mutant p53 protein was demonstrable within surgical specimens in 11/14 (78.5%) patients with cholangiocarcinoma, 10 of whom had undergone liver transplantation and 4 of whom partial liver resection. Tissue from no transplanted patients with long-standing PSC but no evidence of tumour in the explanted liver gave a positive result. The applicability of this approach to the diagnosis of cholangiocarcinoma in clinical practice remains to be determined.

DIFFICULTIES IN PREDICTING WHICH PATIENTS WITH PSC WILL DEVELOP CHOLANGIOCARCINOMA

At least three different studies have purported to identify factors predicting prognosis in PSC. Studies from King's College Hospital[3] and the Mayo Clinic[6] each identified prognostic parameters on the basis of multivariate analysis of large groups of patients from a single centre. In a third study reported by Dickson *et al.*[41], both the Mayo and King's patients were included along with patients from three other centres. Different variables were found as independent indicators of prognosis in these three studies, with only age and the histological stage of PSC common to all. In the King's study, alkaline phosphatase levels and the presence of hepatomegaly and splenomegaly were also considered to influence prognosis, whilst, in the Mayo Clinic series, bilirubin and haemoglobin levels and the presence of IBD were considered important. Bilirubin levels and the presence of splenomegaly were identified as additional prognostic indices in the multicentre study. However, these parameters were considered predictive of overall survival in PSC rather than reflecting the development of cholangiocarcinoma *per se*.

Predicting which PSC patients are at risk of developing cholangiocarcinoma is an important issue in view of the poor prognosis associated with this tumour. The Mayo Clinic series reported by Rosen *et al.*[19] demonstrated median survival from the time of diagnosis of only 5 months (Figure 3), the majority (63%) of patients having evidence of metastatic disease at the time of diagnosis, most commonly to regional lymph nodes. Only one patient was suitable for potentially curative resection and was free of disease 26 months after pancreaticoduodenectomy. The prognosis following liver transplantation in patients with PSC complicated by cholangiocarcinoma is poor, with early tumour recurrence and survival less than two years in most patients[9,10,20,23,28] (Figure 4). In the Pittsburgh series reported by Abu-Elmagd *et al.*[21], median survival was 14 months in those PSC patients in whom cholangiocarcinoma had been diagnosed clinically prior to transplantation and remained only 23 months in those with clinically unsuspected tumour evident in the hepatectomy specimen. Nonetheless, we are currently following one transplant recipient, in whom a clinically unsuspected 3-cm cholangiocarcinoma along with a single lymph node metastasis in the porta hepatis were found in the resected specimen, who has no clinical, biochemical or radiological (including cholangiographic) evidence of tumour recurrence more than eight years later.

Priority clearly needs to be given to developing markers to identify patients who are at high risk of developing cholangiocarcinoma, with a view to liver transplantation before this has occurred. Whilst some authors suggest that cholangiocarcinoma is more likely to develop in patients with end-stage disease[42], most studies indicate that neither age, gender, the presence or absence of pre-existing symptoms, the duration of PSC, the intra- or extrahepatic distribution of PSC, the histological stage of PSC nor the presence or duration of IBD are of predictive value[4,8,9,19,21,22,43]. Conversely, Broome *et al.*[44] have recently reported that cholangiocarcinoma was significantly more prevalent among that subgroup of PSC patients with ulcerative colitis complicated by colorectal dysplasia/carcinoma (7/16, 43.8%) than in those without colorectal neoplasia (2/24, 8.3%). The mean interval between the first detection of the neoplastic lesions in the

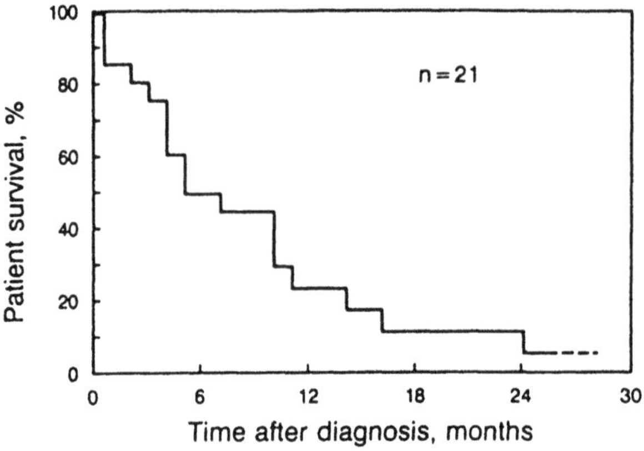

Figure 3 Survival after the diagnosis of primary sclerosing cholangitis (PSC)[19]

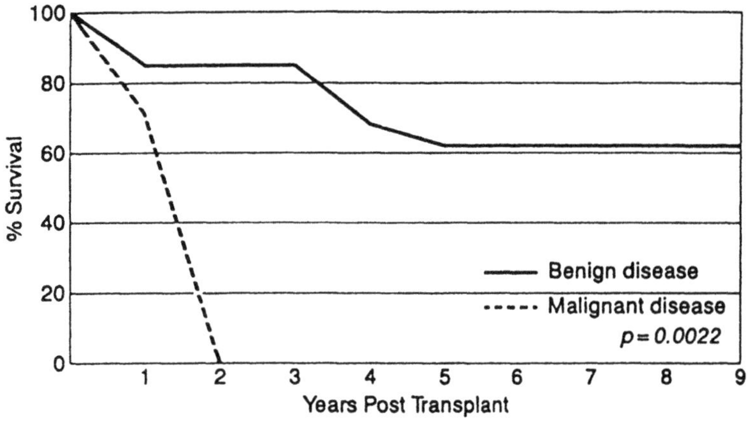

Figure 4 Impact of superimposed cholangiocarcinoma on patient survival in PSC, demonstrated by the absence of survivors beyond 2 years among patients with cholangiocarcinoma who underwent liver transplantation[23]

bowel and the development of cholangiocarcinoma was eight years (range: 0–22 years). If confirmed in other studies, this observation may be of importance when deciding upon the optimal timing of liver transplantation in individual patients with PSC. Martins *et al.*[7] have suggested that the presence of dysplastic biliary epithelium in liver biopsy sections may also be of prognostic significance, based on a patient in whom biliary dysplasia preceded the appearance of cholangiocarcinoma by at least 18 months. However, the possibility of sampling error must be considered, especially in view of the fact that dysplastic biliary epithelium was found away from the tumour area in a second patient, in keeping with other reports of biliary epithelial dysplasia in association with already established cholangiocarcinoma both in the PSC[10] and non-PSC setting[42].

SUMMARY AND CONCLUSIONS

PSC is a premalignant disorder in up to 36% of patients. Despite careful clinical assessment, most tumours arising in this setting are not clinically recognizable and are detected only at autopsy or in the hepatectomy specimens of transplant recipients. This is despite the use of a range of possible screening biochemical tests and imaging techniques. Those cholangiocarcinomas complicating PSC which are diagnosed clinically tend to be detected at an advanced stage, precluding potentially curative surgical resection or liver transplantation. An index based on serum levels of the tumour markers CEA and CA 19-9 has been reported to identify a substantial proportion of PSC patients with otherwise clinically occult cholangiocarcinomas. Whether an increased proportion of tumours identified in this way are amenable to resection remains to be determined. It is doubtful on present evidence whether the outcome following liver transplantation would be improved in such a group, as early tumour recurrence and poor survival have been reported after transplantation in the majority of PSC patients found to have incidental tumours in the hepatectomy specimen. More promising strategies would be designed to reliably identify those individual PSC patients who are at particularly high risk for the development of cholangiocarcinoma, with a view to earlier liver transplantation before the occurrence of tumour in this group. Clinically definable factors, such as age, gender, duration of PSC, the intra- or extrahepatic distribution of PSC and the histological stage of PSC are not of predictive value. Whether the presence of colorectal dysplasia or carcinoma in those patients with both PSC and ulcerative colitis reliably portends future cholangiocarcinoma development, as recently reported, requires further investigation.

References

1. Yee YM, Kaplan MM. Primary sclerosing cholangitis. N Engl J Med. 1995;332:924–33.
2. Weisner RH, LaRusso NF. Clinicopathologic features of the syndrome of primary sclerosing cholangitis. Gastroenterology. 1980;79:200–6.
3. Farrant JM, Hayllar KM, Wilkinson ML *et al.* Natural history and prognostic variables in primary sclerosing cholangitis. Gastroenterology. 1991;100:1710–17.
4. Aadland E, Schrumpf E, Fausa O *et al.* Primary sclerosing cholangitis: a long-term follow-up. Scand J Gastroenterol. 1987;22:655–64.
5. Broome U, Glaumann H, Hellers G, Nilsson B, Sorstad J, Hultcrantz R. Liver disease in ulcerative colitis: an epidemiological and follow up study in the county of Stockholm. Gut. 1994;35: 84–9.
6. Weisner RH, Grambsch PM, Dickson ER *et al.* Primary sclerosing cholangitis: natural history, prognostic factors and survival analysis. Hepatology. 1989;10:430–6.
7. Martins EBG, Fleming KA, Garrido MC, Hine KR, Chapman RWG. Superficial thrombophlebitis, dysplasia and cholangiocarcinoma in primary sclerosing cholangitis. Gastroenterology. 1994;107:537–42.
8. Broome U, Eriksson LS. Assessment for liver transplantation in patients with primary sclerosing cholangitis. J Hepatol. 1994;20:654–9.
9. Marsh JW, Iwatsuki S, Makowka L *et al.* Orthotopic liver transplantation for primary sclerosing cholangitis. Ann Surg. 1988;207:21–5.
10. Miros M, Kerlin P, Walker N, Harper J, Lynch S, Strong R. Predicting cholangiocarcinoma in patients with primary sclerosing cholangitis before transplantation. Gut. 1991;32:1369–73.
11. Schrumpf E, Fausa O, Kolmannskog, Elgjo K, Ritland S, Gjone E. Sclerosing cholangitis in ulcerative colitis: a follow-up study. Scand J Gastroenterol. 1982;17:33–9.

12. Thorpe MEC, Scheuer PJ, Sherlock S. Primary sclerosing cholangitis, the biliary tree and ulcerative colitis. Gut. 1967;8:435–8.
13. Ritchie JK, Allan RN, MacCartney J, Thompson H, Hawley PR, Cooke WT. Biliary tract carcinoma associated with ulcerative colitis. Q J Med. 1974;43:264–8.
14. Mir-Madjlessi SH, Farmer RG, Sivak MV. Bile duct carcinoma in patients with ulcerative colitis. Dig Dis Sci. 1987;32:145–54.
15. Wee A, Ludwig J. Pericholangitis in chronic ulcerative colitis: primary sclerosing cholangitis of the small bile ducts? Ann Intern Med. 1985;102:581–7.
16. Rosen CB, Nagorney DM. Cholangiocarcinoma complicating primary sclerosing cholangitis. Semin Liver Dis. 1991;11:26–30.
17. Chapman RWG, Arborgh BA, Rhodes JM *et al.* Primary sclerosing cholangitis: a review of its clinical features, cholangiography and hepatic histology. Gut. 1980;21:870–7.
18. Lindnor KD, Wiesner RH, MacCarty RL, Ludwig J, LaRusso NF. Advances in primary sclerosing cholangitis. Am J Med. 1990;89:73–80.
19. Rosen CB, Nagorney DM, Wiesner RH, Coffey RJ, LaRusso NF. Cholangiocarcinoma complicating primary sclerosing cholangitis. Ann Surg. 1991;213:21–5.
20. Muiesan P, Shanmugam RP, Devlin J *et al.* Orthotopic liver transplantation for primary sclerosing cholangitis. Transplant Proc. 1994;26:3574–6.
21. Abu-Elmagd KM, Selby R, Iwatsuki S *et al.* Cholangiocarcinoma and sclerosing cholangitis: clinical characteristics and effect on survival after liver transplantation. Transplant Proc. 1993; 25:1124–5.
22. Broome U, Olsson R, Loof L *et al.* Natural history and prognostic factors in 305 Swedish patients with primary sclerosing cholangitis. Gut. 1996;38:610–15.
23. Knechtle SJ, D'Alessandro AM, Harms BA, Pirsch JD, Belzer FO, Kalayoglu M. Relationships between sclerosing cholangitis, inflammatory bowel disease and cancer in patients undergoing liver transplantation. Surgery. 1995;118:615–20.
24. Ismail T, Angrisani L, Powell JE *et al.*. Primary sclerosing cholangitis: surgical options, prognostic variables and outcome. Br J Surg. 1991;78:564–7.
25. Narumi S, Roberts JP, Emond JC, Lake J, Ascher NL. Liver transplantation for sclerosing cholangitis. Hepatology. 1995;22:451–7.
26. Martin FM, Rossi RL, Nugen FW *et al.* Surgical aspects of sclerosing cholangitis. Ann Surg. 1990;212:551–8.
27. Lindnor KD, for the Mayo Primary Sclerosing Cholangitis–Ursodeoxycholic Acid Study Group. Ursodiol for primary sclerosing cholangitis. N Engl J Med. 1996;336:691–5.
28. MacCarty RL, LaRusso NF, May GR *et al.* Cholangiocarcinoma complicating primary sclerosing cholangitis: cholangiographic appearances. Radiology. 1985;156:43–6.
29. Ramage JK, Donaghy A, Farrant JM, Iorns R, Williams R. Serum tumor markers for the diagnosis of cholangiocarcinoma in primary sclerosing cholangitis. Gastroenterology. 1995;108:865–9.
30. Pitt HA, Dooley WC, Yeo CJ, Cameron JL. Malignancies of the biliary tree. Curr Prob Surg. 1995;32:1–100.
31. Mirza DF, Davies M, Olliff S *et al.* Preoperative diagnosis of cholangiocarcinoma in primary sclerosing cholangitis in potential liver transplant candidates. Hepatology. 1994;20:154A.
32. Ferrari-Junior AP, Lichtenstein DR, Slivka A, Chang C, Carr-Locke DL. Brush cytology during ERCP for the diagnosis of biliary and pancreatic malignancies. Gastrointest Endosc. 1994;40: 140–5.
33. Desa LA, Akosa AB, Lazzara S, Domizio P, Krausz T, Benjamin IS. Cytodiagnosis in the management of extrahepatic biliary stricture. Gut. 1991;32:1188–91.
34. Kurzawinski T, Deery A, Dooley J, Dick R, Hobbs K, Davidson B. A prospective controlled study comparing brush and bile exfoliate cytology for diagnosing bile duct stricture. Gut. 1992; 33:1675–7.
35. Rabinovitz M, Zajko AB, Hassanen T *et al.* Diagnostic value of brush cytology in the diagnosis of bile duct carcinoma: a study in 65 patients with bile duct strictures. Hepatology. 1990;12: 747–52.
36. Mansfield JC, Griffin SM, Wadehra V, Matthewson K. A prospective evaluation of cytology from biliary strictures. Gut. 1997;40:671–7.
37. Hall-Craggs MA, Lees WR. Fine needle aspiration biopsy: pancreatic and biliary tumors. AJR. 1986;147:399–403.
38. Nakeeb A, Lipsett PA, Lillemoe KD *et al.* Biliary carcinoembryonic antigen levels are a marker

for cholangiocarcinoma. Am J Surg. 1996;171:147–53.
39. Nichols JC, Gores GJ, LaRusso NF, Wiesner RH, Nagorney DM, Ritts RE. Diagnostic value of serum CA 19-9 for cholangiocarcinoma in patients with primary sclerosing cholangitis. Mayo Clin Proc. 1993;68:874–9.
40. Rizzi PM, Ryder SD, Portmann B, Ramage JK, Naoumov NV, Williams R. p53 protein over-expression in cholangiocarcinoma in primary sclerosing cholangitis. Gut. 1996;38:265–8.
41. Dickson ER, Murtaugh PA, Wiesner RH *et al.* Primary sclerosing cholangitis: refinement and validation of survival models. Gastroenterology. 1992;103:1893–901.
42. Klompmaker IJ, Haagsma EB, Verwer R, Jansen PLM, Slooff MJH. Primary sclerosing cholangitis and liver transplantation. Scand J Gastroenterol. 1996;31,Suppl 218:98–102.
43. Schrumpf E, Abdelnoor M, Fausa O, Elgjo K, Jenssen E, Kolmannskog F. Risk factors in primary sclerosing cholangitis. J Hepatol. 1994;21:1061–6.
44. Broome U, Lofberg R, Veress B, Eriksson LS. Primary sclerosing cholangitis and ulcerative colitis: evidence for increased neoplastic potential. Hepatology. 1995;22:1404–8.

9 Extrahepatic manifestations of primary sclerosing cholangitis

J. NEUBERGER

INTRODUCTION

Although primary sclerosing cholangitis (PSC) is a biliary disease affecting both intrahepatic and extrahepatic bile ducts, there is a strong association with extrahepatic disease, especially with inflammatory bowel disease (IBD). It remains uncertain whether these associations are related to a common cause (such as an infective or environmental trigger), a common factor predisposing to the two conditions (such as HLA), or merely chance (unlikely). In experimental models of colitis in animals, hepatobiliary changes suggestive of PSC can be demonstrated[1]. Familial factors may be involved: one study looking at the familial occurrence of IBD and PSC found three families which had both PSC and UC[2,3]. About 5% of first-degree relatives of patients with PSC (with or without IBD) had PSC, whereas nearly one-third had IBD. These familial occurrences cannot readily differentiate between genetic and environmental factors.

INFLAMMATORY BOWEL DISEASE

The strongest association of PSC with extrahepatic disease is with IBD. The reported frequency of the association varies considerably between series (Table 1). The differences in the reported association may reflect, in part, different methodologies: as discussed below, many patients with PSC may have symptomatically quiescent IBD so that IBD will be detected only if colonoscopy is done and biopsies taken; conversely, the presence of an elevated serum alkaline phosphatase in a patient with IBD does not necessarily mean the patient has PSC; for example, other liver diseases such as chronic hepatitis are associated with IBD and the elevated serum alkaline phosphatase may be due to intestinal or bone disease. As can be seen from Tables 1 and 2, the reported associations will depend on whether the series is reported from a clinic looking after patients with IBD or with liver disease. Thus, while only a relatively small number of patients

Table 1 Occurrence of PSC in patients with UC

Reference	*n*	*Percentage*
Schrumpf *et al.*[40]	336	7.5
Sheppard *et al.*[41]	681	2.4
Tobias *et al.*[42]	250	3

Table 2 Occurrence of IBD in patients with PSC

Reference	*PSC (n)*	*Percentage IBD*	*Percentage UC*	*Percentage CD*
Helzberg *et al.*[9]	53	62	94	6
Takikawa and Manabe[5]	192	21	95	5
Wiesner *et al.*[8]	174	71	n/a	n/a
Rabinowitz *et al.*[9]	66	71	83	17
Okada *et al.*[10]	155	23	84	–
Fausa *et al.*[43]	60	98	80	14
Broome *et al.*[44]	305	81	72	7
Okolicsanyi *et al.*[45]	117	54	67	–

Series of >50 patients only included. PSC = primary sclerosing cholangitis, UC = ulcerative colitis, CD = Crohn's disease. The totals do not always add up to 100% since, in some series, patients had other forms of bowel disease

with ulcerative colitis have PSC, approximately three-quarters of patients with PSC have some type of IBD.

One of the features apparent from Table 2 is that the two reports from Japan show a much lower prevalence of IBD in patients with PSC than do studies from Europe and North America. Okada *et al.*[4] compared a Japanese series of patients with PSC with data from several European and North American centres. Japanese PSC patients with IBD tended to be younger (mean age 33 compared with 52 years in those without IBD), were more likely to be female (51% compared with 36%). As with European/North American series, most of the patients (74%) had extensive colitis which was usually diagnosed prior to the diagnosis of PSC. Takikawa and Manabe[5] reached similar conclusions, based on a postal questionnaire sent to members of the Japanese Society of Gastroenterology. There are clearly limitations with such an approach. Why the association of PSC and IBD is so much lower in Japan remains unclear. Whether these differences can be accounted for merely by differences in diagnostic criteria, in referral patterns or assessment is uncertain; alternatively, this difference may relate to host factors (such as HLA) or environmental causes. Identification of the reasons for the difference will be of value in understanding the relationship of the two diseases.

In general, PSC and IBD are diagnosed at the same time, or IBD has been present for a decade or more before the PSC is diagnosed. The routine availability of liver function tests has increased the awareness of coexisting, asymptomatic liver disease, and the routine use of endoscopic biliary imaging has made the diagnosis of PSC much easier. The increasing power of magnetic resonance imaging is likely to make a non-invasive diagnosis of PSC easy. However, it is well recognized that PSC may be diagnosed several years after proctocolectomy; thus PSC can be diagnosed before, during or after the diagnosis of IBD.

It has been suggested that the association of PSC with IBD may identify a variant of PSC[6]: the median age at diagnosis of PSC is 40 years and males are more likely to develop the condition than females. Rabinovitz *et al.*[7] found a lower male to female ratio in those with PSC and without IBD (0.77:1) compared to those with IBD (2.9:1).

There are conflicting data as to whether all patients with PSC will develop IBD[6]; the data from Scandinavia suggest that all patients in time will develop IBD, while the data from England and North America suggest that only three-quarters will. Reasons for this discrepancy are not clear and may relate, in part, to referral patterns or to methods of diagnosis.

There are conflicting data as to whether the coexistence of IBD affects the prognosis and progression of PSC: studies from the Mayo Clinic[8] suggested that PSC patients with concomitant IBD had a worse prognosis than those without IBD; these findings have not been confirmed by others[9]. However, it is difficult to disentangle the effects of the two diseases on the mode and place of presentation. The hepatic histological features are similar in those with and without IBD.

PSC AND ULCERATIVE COLITIS

The pattern of colonic disease activity in patients with ulcerative colitis (UC) appears to be different in those with and without PSC. Lundqvist and Broome[10], in a retrospective study, compared the clinical course of 29 patients with PSC and total colitis each with two matched controls without PSC. The observation period was over 20 years. Compared with patients with UC alone, there was a similar sex ratio (72% compared with 62% males). There was no difference between patients in the two groups in those taking prophylactic therapy, those with UC alone received treatment with topical and with systemic corticosteroids significantly more often than those with PSC and UC: thus, of those with UC and PSC, 58% and 52% had not been treated with local or systemic corticosteroids, compared with 28% and 24% respectively for those with UC alone. Equally, hospitalization for colonic disease was required significantly more often for those with UC alone. However, there was no difference between the groups with respect to the proportion with continuous colitis. In contrast, colectomy was undertaken in 11 (38%) of patients with PSC (for prophylactic reasons (one), disease activity (three) and dysplasia (seven)) compared with 11 (19%) of those with UC alone (disease activity (four) and dysplasia (seven)).

Whilst these observations suggest that the disease activity in those with PSC and UC is less, there is the potential for bias, since those with mild colitis might not be referred to a specialist IBD clinic. There are obvious concerns that this is a retrospective study, but the likelihood for bias is small.

That the colonic activity in patients with PSC differs from that in those without the PSC is further supported by observations from Penna and colleagues[11] who studied the extent of pouchitis in patients after ileo-anal pouch anastomosis. The records of 1097 patients who had undergone ileal pouch–anal anastomosis were studied; of these patients, just 54 (5%) had coincident PSC. Pouchitis was documented by clinical, endoscopic and histological criteria. Pouchitis developed in 32% of those without coincident PSC and in 63% of those with PSC. The 1, 2, 5 and 10 year probability of developing pouchitis in those without PSC was 15.5%, 22.5%, 36% and 45.5% and for those with PSC the retrospective cumulative risks were 22%, 43%, 61% and 79%. Thus, in those with PSC, pouchitis occurs earlier and more frequently. Multivariate analysis suggests that the presence of PSC is an independent risk factor for the development of pouchitis. These findings confirm earlier results from the same group[12]. The implications of these observations for the pathogenesis of PSC or pouchitis are not clear: whether pouchitis represents recurrent UC, the effects of other factors such as altered bile acid pool, ischaemia, nutritional deficiency, a local toxic factor or involvement of immune mechanisms, is not clear.

Despite the risks of pouchitis developing in patients with PSC, Penna and colleagues still recommend the construction of a pouch in patients with UC requiring a colectomy; the experience at the Mayo Clinic[13] was that, of patients with PSC who underwent a proctocolectomy and Brooke's ileostomy, peristomal varices developed in more than half, and were often associated with troublesome stomal variceal haemorrhage. Our own limited experience has found a lower incidence of stomal variceal development, and such variceal bleeding can be controlled readily by the use of a transjugular intrahepatic portosystemic shunt (TIPSS).

UC AFTER LIVER TRANSPLANTATION

As suggested above, the reasons for the association between PSC and ulcerative colitis are still unclear. However, replacing the PSC liver does not prevent the development of UC after transplantation of the liver, even though these patients are receiving immunosuppression. Riley and colleagues[14] described 14 patients who developed IBD after liver or kidney transplantation. Cases were identified retrospectively from the records of 6800 transplant recipients; few conclusions can be drawn from this analysis about the incidence or prevalence of IBD after transplantation. Of these 14 patients, 12 had undergone liver transplantation and only two were grafted for PSC; of interest, one other was grafted for biliary atresia. Since occurrence of PSC in the graft may occur, these observations do not exclude a causal relationship between the two conditions.

COMPARISON OF PATIENTS WITH UC WITH AND WITHOUT PSC

As is clear from the above discussion, patients with UC and PSC seem to have a different clinical pattern of colonic disease compared with those who have UC alone. There are other clinical features, some of which may point to an explanation of the association. However, it may be difficult to distinguish those abnormalities which arise as a consequence of the liver disease rather than the cause: thus the effect of biliary antigen in inhibiting *in-vitro* leucocyte responses of patients with PSC and UC, and not of those with UC alone, may be a consequence of the bile duct damage[15]; similarly, impaired clearance of immune complexes seen in patients with PSC and UC, but not in those with UC alone, may also reflect a degree of liver damage[16].

However, as described in greater detail elsewhere in this volume, Chapman[17] and Zauli *et al.*[18] have reported a different pattern of autoantibodies in patients with PSC and UC. Of greater significance, there are differences in HLA genotypes. Thus there is a high proportion of HLA Drw52a in patients with PSC[19], whether or not they have UC, whereas the association with UC is less clear, possibly with B8, B27 and Bw25[20].

PSC AND CROHN'S DISEASE

While PSC is usually associated with UC, some cases are associated with Crohn's disease (Table 2). Rasmussen and colleagues from Aalborg recently reported their experience of hepatobiliary dysfunction in patients with Crohn's disease[21]. They studied 262 patients with Crohn's disease over a 15-year period. Of these patients, 38 (15%) had elevation of serum alkaline phosphatase, between 321 and 4165 IU/L (mean 1065 IU/L). Of these, 10 patients were found to have hepatobiliary diseases: nine had PSC, confirmed by imaging the biliary tree and by liver biopsy, and one a non-specific reactive hepatitis. Of these nine patients with PSC, the disease affected the large ducts in three, the small ducts in five (that is to say the ERCP was normal) and one was unclassified. In the 102 patients in their series with large bowel Crohn's disease, the incidence of PSC was 9%. Two of these patients developed colonic carcinoma. The male:female ratio was 2:7. The liver disease was at a relatively early stage, with all those with small bile duct PSC at histological stage 1, whereas in those with large duct PSC, the stages were 2 and 3. The authors suggest that those with PSC and Crohn's disease may have milder liver disease than those with PSC and UC, but caution must be used in extrapolating from relatively small numbers. Furthermore, there has been some doubt over the significance of 'small duct PSC', which may be similar to the older term of pericholangitis[22]. However, Lee and Ludwig described two cases who developed large duct PSC some time after being diagnosed as having small duct disease, indicating that the two conditions represent a spectrum[23].

Where PSC is linked to Crohn's disease it is almost invariably to large bowel, and the extent of colonic involvement is likely to be extensive.

PSC, UC AND COLONIC NEOPLASIA

Patients with PSC are at risk of developing cholangiocarcinoma; indeed, it is argued that PSC is a premalignant condition. In 1992 Broome and colleagues suggested that PSC itself was an independent risk factor for the development of colonic dysplasia[24]. In a subsequent study[46] they used a retrospective case-record analysis to determine the cumulative risk of colorectal neoplasia in patients with PSC and UC: 40 patients with extensive UC and with PSC were matched each with two patients with UC but without PSC; matching was according to age, extent and duration of colitis. All patients with UC were under colonic surveillance, with endoscopies and biopsies. Among the 40 patients with PSC and UC, colonic neoplasia and/or cancer developed in 16 patients, compared with 10 of 80 in the group with UC alone. The cumulative risk of developing colorectal cancer/dysplasia at 10, 20 and 25 years was 9%, 31% and 50% in those with PSC and UC, compared with 2%, 5% and 10% respectively in those with UC alone.

Several other groups have also examined whether the presence of PSC is associated with an increased risk of colonic neoplasia. Brentnall *et al.*[25] followed 20 patients with PSC and UC and 25 comparison patients with UC alone, using regular colonoscopy and multiple biopsies. Whereas nine of the 20 (45%) patients with PSC and UC developed colonic dysplasia, only four of the 25 (16%) of the control patients did so. None of the patients in this study developed colon cancer. One confounding factor in this study was that five of the patients with PSC had undergone liver transplantation: of these three had dysplasia and one had indefinite dysplasia. Liver transplantation (and presumably the consequent immunosuppression) is associated with an increased risk of colonic carcinoma, even in patients grafted for indications other than PSC and without IBD[26]. When logistic regression analysis was used to define those factors which are associated with the development of colonic dysplasia, three factors were identified:

1. presence of primary sclerosing cholangitis,
2. duration of disease,
3. age of onset of UC.

Only the presence of PSC was significantly associated with colonic dysplasia ($p = 0.002$).

Other studies have also suggested an increased risk of colonic neoplasia in patients with PSC: thus, D'Haens and colleagues in Chicago[27] reported an increased cancer risk in patients with PSC and pericholangitis, although these entities were poorly defined and there were concerns about the possible referral bias and population size[28]. A retrospective case-note study from the Veterans Hospital found a significant association between sclerosing cholangitis[29], and Gurbuz and colleagues[30] found an incidence of colorectal dysplasia or cancer in 13 of 35 (13%), although the cumulative incidence of cancer was similar to an historical control group with pancolitis.

An initial study from the Mayo Clinic[31] failed to find any evidence of an increased risk of colonic neoplasia in PSC: a sample of 178 patients were stratified by area of residence, and the relative risk of colonic cancer estimated using age- and sex-specific incidence rates, using data both from patients with UC in central Sweden and in the US general population. Of the 178 patients, 77% had a colitis, which involved the entire colon in 74%. Colorectal cancer was diagnosed in eight patients: three prior and five after the diagnosis of PSC was made. The site of the cancer was caecum (one), transverse colon (two), splenic flexure (one), descending colon (three) and sigmoid (one). Although there was an increased risk of colon cancer in these patients compared with the general, matched population, there were no excess cancers compared to patients with UC alone. Proportional hazards regression analysis did not identify any risk factor for the development of colonic cancer. An accompanying editorial[32] discussed the possible reasons for the apparent conflict in conclusions. Ahnen[32] drew attention to differences in design, choice of end-points, problems in execution and interpretation and, in particular, the control group.

However, a subsequent report from the Mayo Clinic[33] reached similar conclusions, using a different approach to analysis. A total of 203 patients with UC and colorectal cancer diagnosed at the Clinic between 1976 and 1994 were identified.

Controls (199 patients) were UC patients without evidence of dysplasia or cancer, diagnosed during the same period and matched for age, sex, duration and extent of colitis. There was a similar proportion of patients with PSC in the two groups (34 (18%) in those with colorectal cancer and 27 (14%) in the comparison group). A logistic regression model again found no evidence of PSC as a risk factor for colorectal cancer (adjusted odds ratio 1.3 (95% confidence limits 0.72–2.37)).

However, other series have suggested an increased risk of colon cancer in patients with PSC: Marchesa and colleagues[34] evaluated 1212 patients who had undergone a total proctocolectomy with the formation of an ileal pouch–anal anastomosis. Of these, 27 had PSC and were compared with the remaining patients. Dysplasia, detected during routine surveillance, was the indication for colectomy in 18 (67%) of those with PSC and in only 142 (12%) of those without PSC, thus the relative risk of PSC for colonic dysplasia is 5.5 (95% CI 3.7–8.3). Pathological examination of the resected specimen showed cancer in 15% of those with PSC and only in 4% of the comparison group (RR 3.6, CI 1.4–9.1). All four patients with PSC had the cancer located in the right side of the colon (proximal to the splenic flexure) compared with 41% of the comparison group. Leidenius *et al.*[35] also evaluated the effect of PSC on the colon cancer risk in IBD: the clinical courses of 45 patients with PSC and UC were matched with 45 controls with UC alone. Thirteen (29%) of those with PSC and UC developed colorectal neoplasia (carcinoma (four), high-grade dysplasia (two) and low-grade dysplasia (seven)). In contrast, four (9%) of the comparison patients developed neoplastic findings (carcinoma (one), high-grade dysplasia (one), low-grade dysplasia (two)).

Because of the conflict within the literature, Soetkino and colleagues[36] undertook a meta-analysis of studies, identified by Medline analysis, manual searches and contacting relevant authors directly. They concluded that patients with UC and PSC have an increased risk of colorectal neoplasia compared to those with UC alone: odds ratio of 3.68 (95% CI 2.55–5.29); when the analysis was restricted to carcinoma alone, PSC remained a significant risk factor, OR 3.20 (95% CI 2.08–4.88).

Thus, on balance, it appears that the presence of PSC is associated with an increased risk of colorectal cancer compared with those with ulcerative colitis alone. The finding of an increase in right-sided cancers has led to the suggestion that the presence of abnormal bile pool in the colon may be important. However, there may be other factors, such as immunological or genetic, which may play a role. Furthermore, because the course of colitis in patients with PSC differs from that in those with UC alone, it is possible that methodological factors may play a part in the reported increased risk.

IMPLICATIONS OF IBD IN THE MANAGEMENT OF PATIENTS WITH PSC

The above findings suggest that:

1. All patients with PSC should undergo full colonoscopic examination at diagnosis, and that biopsies should be taken even in the presence of normal

macroscopic appearance. Barium studies and flexible sigmoidoscopy are inadequate to diagnose the presence and extent of colitis.

2. If colitis is present, then these patients should be considered for inclusion in a cancer surveillance programme, with attention paid to the proximal as well as distal colon.
3. If dysplasia or cancer is present, a colectomy should be done; the formation of an ileostomy may be associated with stomal varices which may cause problematic haemorrhage.
4. Colitis should be treated in the conventional way, although relatively few will require additional topical or systemic corticosteroids.
5. The risks and complications of colitis remain after liver transplantation.

OTHER EXTRAHEPATIC FEATURES

There have been many other conditions associated with PSC; some of these are associated with the same HLA genotype as PSC, others may represent little more than a coincidence (Table 3).

The commoner associations of PSC are with pancreatitis, which may be present in up to 15% of patients. Imaging the pancreatic duct may show enlargement suggestive of malignancy; cannulation of the pancreatic duct shows the inflammatory changes. Pohl and Junge[37] reported one case in whom there was an excellent clinical response to ursodeoxycholic acid, and substitution of the endocrine and exocrine functions of the pancreas. It should be remembered that azathioprine, often used in the management of UC, can cause pancreatitis. The association between PSC, fibrosing pancreatitis and other fibrosing conditions suggests that there may be common underlying mechanisms, and perhaps some extraneous factor results in damage to one or more organs. It is important for the clinician to be aware of the associated diseases: thus, weight loss should not necessarily be attributed to the progression of liver disease, but other factors should be considered.

Sarcoidosis is well recognized to be associated with PSC and occurs in less than 1%[38]. A retrospective study from the Mayo Clinic identified 10 cases among

Table 3 Extrahepatic conditions reported to be associated with PSC

Coeliac sprue	Retroperitoneal fibrosis
Biliary atresia	Thyroiditis
Polymyositis	Sjögren's syndrome
Alopecia	Systemic lupus
Haemolytic anaemia	Vasculitis
Dermatitis herpetiformis	Peyronie's disease
Pancreatitis	Bronchiectasis
Rheumatoid arthritis	Cystic fibrosis
Nephropathy	Eosinophilic syndrome
Membranous nephropathy	Diabetes mellitus
Thyrotoxicosis	Histiocytosis X
Sarcoidosis	

1401 cases of PSC. Seven of the 10 had UC; sarcoidosis was diagnosed at about the same age as the PSC, although UC was detected 10 years earlier. Eight patients had a hilar lymphadenopathy and six interstitial lung disease. Liver, bone marrow and ocular involvement was present in one patient each. An elevated level of serum angioconverting enzyme was present in only half of those with sarcoidosis. There is an association with the HLA phenotypes B8 and DR3. Sarcoidosis can occur in both UC and in Crohn's disease in the absence of liver disease[39].

References

1. Wojszys R. Liver involvement and its course in experimental colitis in rats. Hepatogastroenterology. 1997;44:1193–5.
2. Quigley E. Familial occurrence of primary sclerosing cholangitis and ulcerative colitis. Gastroenterology. 1983;85:1160–5.
3. Jorge AD, Esley C, Ahumada J. Family incidence of primary sclerosing cholangitis associated with immunological diseases. Endoscopy. 1987;19:114–17.
4. Okada H, Mizuno M, Amamoto K, Tsuji T. Primary sclerosing cholangitis in Japanese patients – association with inflammatory bowel disease. Acta Med Okayama. 1996;50:227–35.
5. Takikawa H, Manabe T. Primary sclerosing cholangitis in Japan – analysis of 192 cases. J Gastroenterol. 1997;32:134–7.
6. Fausa O, Schrumpf E, Elgjo K. Relationship of inflammatory bowel disease and primary sclerosing cholangitis. Semin Liver Dis. 1991;11:31–9.
7. Rabinovitz M, Gavaler J, Schade R *et al.* Does primary sclerosing cholangitis occurring in association with inflammatory bowel disease differ from that occurring in the absence of inflammatory bowel disease? A study of sixty-six subjects. Hepatology. 1990;11:7–11.
8. Wiesner RH, Grambsch P, Dickson ER *et al.* Primary sclerosing cholangitis: natural history, prognostic factors and survival analysis. Histology. 1989;10:430–6.
9. Helzberg JH, Petersen J, Boyer J. Improved survival with primary sclerosing cholangitis: a review of clinicopathologic features and comparison of symptomatic and asymptomatic patients. Gastroenterology. 1987;92:1869–75.
10. Lundqvist K, Broome U. Differences in colonic disease activity in patients with ulcerative colitis with and without primary sclerosing cholangitis. Dis Colon Rectum. 1997;40:451–6.
11. Penna C, Dozois R, Tremaine W *et al.* Pouchitis after ileal pouch–anal anastomosis for ulcerative colitis occurs with increased frequency in patients with associated primary sclerosing cholangitis. Gut. 1996;38:234–9.
12. Kartheuser AH, Dozois RR, Wiesner R, La Russo N, Ilstrup DM, Schleck CD. Complications and risk factors after ileal pouch–anal anastomosis for ulcerative colitis associated with primary sclerosing cholangitis. Ann Surg. 1993;217:314–20.
13. Wiesner R, La Russo N, Dozois R, Beaver S. Peristomal varices after proctocolectomy in patients with primary sclerosing cholangitis. Gastroenterology. 1986;90:316–22.
14. Riley T, Schoen R, Lee RG, Rakela J. A case series of transplant recipients who despite immunosuppression developed inflammatory bowel disease. Am J Gastroenterol. 1998;92:279–82.
15. McFarlane IG, Wojcicka B, Tsantoulas D, Eddleston E, Portmann B, Williams R. Leucocyte migration inhibition in response to biliary antigens in primary biliary cirrhosis, sclerosing cholangitis and other chronic liver diseases. Gastroenterology. 1979;76:1333–40.
16. Minuk G, Hershfield N, Lee W. Reticuloendothelial system Fc receptor-mediated clearance of IgG-tagged erythrocytes from the circulation of patients with ulcerative colitis and chronic liver disease. Hepatology. 1986;6:1–5.
17. Chapman R, Cottone M, Selby W, Sherlock S. Serum autoantibodies, ulcerative colitis and primary sclerosing cholangitis. Gut. 1986;27:86–91.
18. Zauli D, Schrumpf E, Crespi C *et al.* An autoantibody profile in primary sclerosing cholangitis. J Hepatol. 1987;5:14–18.
19. Donaldson P, Farrant M, Wilkinson M, Hayllar K, Portmann B, Williams R. Dual association of HLADR2 and DR3 with primary sclerosing cholangitis. Hepatology. 1991;13:129–33.
20. Hodgson H, Jewell D. Inflammatory bowel disease. Bailliere's Clin Gastroenterol. 1987;1:

531–45.
21. Rasmussen HH, Fallingborg J, Mortensen P, Vyberg M, Tage Jensen U, Rasmussen S. Hepatobiliary dysfunction and primary sclerosing cholangitis in patients with Crohn's disease. Scand J Gastroenterol. 1997;32:604–10.
22. Lee Y-M, Kaplan M. Primary sclerosing cholangitis. N Engl J Med. 1995;332:924–33.
23. Lee A, Ludwig J. Pericholangitis in chronic ulcerative colitis: primary sclerosing cholangitis of the small ducts? Ann Intern Med. 1985;102:581–7.
24. Broome U, Lindberg G, Lofberg R. Primary sclerosing cholangitis, a risk factor for the development of dysplasia and DNA aneuploidy? Gastroenterology. 1992;102:1877–80.
25. Brentall T, Haggitt R, Rabinovitch P *et al.* Risk and natural history of colonic neoplasia in patients with primary sclerosing cholangitis and ulcerative colitis. Gastroenterology. 1996;110: 331–8.
26. Polson R, Neuberger J, Forman D, Calne R, Williams R. De novo malignancy after liver transplantation. Transplant Proc. 1988;20:94–7.
27. D'Haens GR, Lashner BA, Hanauer S. Pericholangitis and sclerosing cholangitis are risk factors for dysplasia and cancer in ulcerative colitis. Am J Gastroenterol. 1993;88:1174–8.
28. Levine D. Pericholangitis in patients with ulcerative colitis, and risk factors for progression to colorectal cancer. Am J Gastroenterol. 1993;88:1151–4.
29. Bansal P, Sonnenberg A. Sclerosing cholangitis as a risk factor for gastrointestinal cancer. Gastroenterology. 1995;108:A405 (abstract).
30. Gurbuz AK, Giardello FM, Bayless TM. Colorectal neoplasia in patients with ulcerative colitis and primary sclerosing cholangitis. Dis Colon Rectum. 1995;38:37–41.
31. Loftus E, Sandborn W, Tremaine W *et al.* Risk of colorectal neoplasia in patients with primary sclerosing cholangitis. Gastroenterology. 1996;110:432–40.
32. Ahnen A. Controlled clinical trials: the controls are the key. Gastroenterology. 1996;110:628–42.
33. Nuako K, Ahlquist D, Siems D, Mahoney D, Sandborn W, Zinsmeister A. Primary sclerosing cholangitis (PSC) as a risk factor for colorectal cancer in ulcerative colitis: a case–control study. Gastroenterology. 1996;110:A981 (abstract).
34. Marchesa P, Fazio V, Lavery I *et al.* The risk of cancer and dysplasia among ulcerative colitis patients with primary sclerosing cholangitis. Gastroenterology. 1996;110:A956 (abstract).
35. Leidenius M, Farkkila M, Farkkainen P, Taskinen E, Kellokumpu I, Hockerstedt K. Colorectal dysplasia and carcinoma in patients with ulcerative colitis and primary sclerosing cholangitis. Scand J Gastroenterol. 1997;32:706–11.
36. Soetkino R, Heidrenreich P, Young H, Blackstone M. Increased risk of colorectal neoplasia in patients with primary sclerosing cholangitis and ulcerative colitis. Gastroenterology. 1997;112: A43 (abstract).
37. Pohl R, Junge U. Primary sclerosing cholangitis with chronic pancreatitis. Deutsche Med Wochenschr. 1997;122:778–82.
38. Joseph JK, Porayko M, Steers J *et al.* The association of primary sclerosing cholangitis and sarcoidosis. Gastroenterology. 1996;110:A1224 (abstract).
39. Fries W, Grassi S, Leone L *et al.* Association between inflammatory bowel disease and sarcoidosis – report of two cases and review of the literature. Scand J Gastroenterol. 1995;30: 1221–3.
40. Schrumpf E, Elgjo K, Fausa O *et al.* Sclerosing cholangitis in ulcerative colitis. Scand J Gastroenterol. 1980;15:689–90.
41. Shepherd H, Selby W, Chapman RWG *et al.* Ulcerative colitis and persistent liver dysfunction. Q J Med. 1983;52:503–13.
42. Tobias R, Wright J, Kottler RE *et al.* Primary sclerosing cholangitis associated with inflammatory bowel disease in Cape Town. S Afr J Med. 1983;63:229–35.
43. Fausa O, Schrumpf E, Elgjo K. Inflammatory bowel disease occurs in almost all patients with primary sclerosing cholangitis. Scand J Gastroenterol. 1989;23:53.
44. Broome U, Glaumann H, Hellers G, Sorstad J, Nillson B, Hultcrantz R. Liver disease in ulcerative colitis: an epidemiological and follow-up study in the county of Stockholm. Gut. 1994;35:84–9.
45. Okolicsanyi L, Fabris L, Viaggi S, Carulli N, Podda M, Ricci G and the Italian PSC Study Group. Primary sclerosing cholangitis: clinical presentation, natural history and prognostic variables: an Italian multi-centre study. Eur J Gastroenterol Hepatol. 1996;8:685–91.
46. Broome U, Lofberg R, Veress B, Eriksson E. Primary sclerosing cholangitis and ulcerative colitis: evidence for increased neoplastic potential. Hepatology. 1995;1404–8.

Section III
Non-surgical treatment

10
Treatment of primary sclerosing cholangitis: the role of ursodeoxycholic acid and endoscopy

A. STIEHL, C. BENZ, P. SAUER and L. THEILMANN

Attempts to treat patients with primary sclerosing cholangitis (PSC) with immunosuppressive, anti-inflammatory or antifibrotic agents were not very successful. Since repeated episodes of bacterial cholangitis are typical for the disease, immunosuppressive treatment may even be harmful. The major breakthrough came with the observation that ursodeoxycholic acid (UDCA) has a beneficial effect on patients with primary biliary cirrhosis (PBC). Subsequently, patients with various forms of cholestatic liver disease, including PSC, have been treated with UDCA[1–5]. A problem arises since the stenoses of the major bile ducts cannot be treated with UDCA and require endoscopic treatment[6–14].

EFFECT OF UDCA ON LABORATORY PARAMETERS

In 1987, we started a trial in patients with PSC[1]. After a 1-year treatment period with UDCA which showed beneficial effects similar to those in PBC and good tolerance in patients with additional ulcerative colitis, a double-blind placebo-controlled study was initiated. UDCA led to significant improvement of AP, GGT, ALT and AST. Serum cholesterol decreased in patients with elevated levels before treatment and was unchanged in the others[1]. Changes in IgA, IgM and IgG were not significant. The changes are similar to those in three other controlled studies (Table 1) in which, in contrast to our study, serum bilirubin also improved significantly[2,4,5].

In a further controlled study in which a relatively low dose of UDCA (600 mg/day) was used, no improvement in laboratory parameters was observed[3], indicating that such a low dose is ineffective and 10–15 mg/day of UDCA should be given.

Table 1 UDCA in PSC: results of placebo-controlled studies[a]

Authors	*n*	*AP, GGT, ALT or AST*	*Bilirubin*	*Histology*
Stiehl *et al.*[1,6]	20	Improved	Unchanged	Favourable[b]
Beuers *et al.*[2]	14	Improved	Improved	Favourable
Lindor *et al.*[4]	105	Improved	Improved	–
Mitchell *et al.*[5]	24	Improved	Improved	Favourable

[a]Studies with UDCA doses >10 mg/kg. [b]Favourable effect in comparison with pretreatment histology

EFFECT OF UDCA ON SYMPTOMS

The effect of UDCA on symptoms is small. Approximately one third of our patients with PSC suffered from pruritus and one half from fatigue[1]. During treatment with UDCA, both symptoms improved in some of the patients but, in comparison with placebo, the effect was not significant.

EFFECT OF UDCA ON LIVER HISTOLOGY

Since PSC is a focal disease, evaluation of liver histology is difficult. In the 3 studies in which the changes in liver histology were evaluated after UDCA treatment, cellular infiltrates in the portal triads decreased significantly whereas all other changes were not significant[1,2,6]. In the Mayo study, no effect of UDCA treatment on liver histology has been reported[4]. A decrease in portal inflammation after UDCA has also been observed in patients with PBC. It is unclear at present whether a decrease of the inflammation around the bile ducts in PSC will have an effect on the development of bile duct carcinomas in this disease.

ENDOSCOPIC TREATMENT OF STENOSES OF MAJOR BILE DUCTS

Several reports exist on the endoscopic treatment of major duct stenoses in PSC (Table 2). In our series, endoscopic balloon dilatation was the preferred form of treatment[6]. After the end of a controlled study period, all our patients were enrolled in a prospective trial on the effect of UDCA on bile duct disease in which repeat cholangiographies were performed[6]. During treatment with UDCA of 65 patients treated for up to 8 years (mean 45 months), 10 developed progressive stenoses of major bile ducts. Endoscopic dilatation of these stenoses is highly effective[6–14]. Repeat cholangiography in patients with narrowing of major bile ducts seems to be essential to detect stenoses of major bile ducts early[6]. It is evident that mechanical obstruction of major bile ducts cannot be treated by UDCA effectively and that endoscopic measures are essential if conservative treatment is to be effective.

Table 2 Endoscopic treatment of patients with PSC with dominant stenoses of major bile ducts

Authors	*Number of patients*	*Stents (n)*	*Dilatations (n)*
Johnson *et al.*[8]	35	11	24
Cotton *et al.*[13]	53	22	31
Huitbregtse *et al.*[14]	25	21	0
Stiehl *et al.*[6]	28	5	91

BILE DUCT CARCINOMA

An unresolved problem in the treatment of patients with PSC is the development of bile duct carcinomas. In a large multicentre study from Sweden, in which 305 PSC patients were followed over a median follow-up time of 63 months, a bile duct carcinoma was observed in 8% of patients and 44% of these were asymptomatic at the time of diagnosis of PSC[15]. In 37% of the patients with bile duct carcinoma, this diagnosis was made within 1 year after detection of PSC and, as a consequence, it seems possible that the patients already had a bile duct carcinoma when the PSC was recognized. This study, at present, represents the largest series available and no factors were found which would allow the identification of patients who will later develop a bile duct carcinoma.

The 8% carcinomas in the Swedish multicentre study is similar to the figure reported by others[16–20] and appears to be much lower than that observed at the Mayo Clinic[21]. Very high rates of bile duct carcinomas have repeatedly been reported in studies from transplantation centres and it appears that they reflect very selected patient groups. In patients treated with UDCA, 3% developed a bile duct carcinoma[6]. It is unclear at present whether UDCA treatment can reduce the incidence of bile duct carcinomas.

SURVIVAL

The findings of a recent controlled 2-year study[4], in which endoscopic treatment of major duct stenoses 'did not play a role', indicate that UDCA treatment does not improve survival free of liver transplantation. This is in contrast to a prospective non-randomized study, in which, from May 1987 up to December 1995, 65 patients were treated with UDCA and, whenever necessary, with additional endoscopic dilatations. The actuarial Kaplan Meier estimate of survival after treatment with UDCA and dilatation of major duct stenoses was significantly improved compared with the predicted survival[6], with $p = 0.001$. The study is ongoing and we hope that this prospective study, with more than 80 patients, will bring additional information on the long-term incidence of bile duct and colonic carcinomas of patients treated with UDCA and also on the long-term survival free of liver transplantation.

CONCLUSION

We conclude that PSC may be treated conservatively by UDCA with good treatment results and prolongation of survival free of liver transplantation only when patients who develop major duct stenoses are recognized early and are treated by endoscopic means. In endstage disease, liver transplantation is indicated.

References

1. Stiehl A, Walker S, Stiehl L *et al.* Effects of ursodeoxycholic acid on liver and bile duct disease in primary sclerosing cholangitis. A 3 year pilot study with a placebo-controlled study period. J Hepatol. 1994;20:57–64.
2. Beuers U, Spengler U, Kruis W *et al.* Ursodeoxycholic acid for treatment of primary sclerosing cholangitis: a placebo controlled trial. Hepatology. 1992;16:707–14.
3. De Maria N, Colantoni A, Rosenblom E, Van Thiel DH. Ursodeoxycholic acid does not improve the clinical course of primary sclerosing cholangitis over a 2-year period. Hepato-Gastroenterology. 1996;43:1472–9.
4. Lindor KD and the Mayo PSC/UDCA Study Group. Ursodiol for the treatment of primary sclerosing cholangitis. N Engl J Med. 1997;336:691–5.
5. Mitchell SA, Bansi D, Hunt N *et al.* High dose ursodeoxycholic acid (UDCA) in primary sclerosing cholangitis (PSC): results after two years of a randomized double-blind, placebo-controlled trial. Abstract. Gut. 1997;40(Suppl.1):TH 115.
6. Stiehl A, Rudolph G, Sauer P *et al.* Efficacy of ursodeoxycholic acid and endoscopic dilation of major duct stenoses in primary sclerosing cholangitis. An 8-year prospective study. J Hepatol. 1997;26:560–6.
7. Grijm R, Huibregtse K, Bartelsman J *et al.* Therapeutic investigations in primary sclerosing cholangitis. Dig Dis Sci. 1986;31:792–8.
8. Johnson GK, Geenen JE, Venu RP, Hogan WJ. Endoscopic treatment of biliary duct strictures in sclerosing cholangitis: Follow up assessment of a new therapeutic approach. Gastrointest Endosc. 1987;33:9–12.
9. Huitbregtse K. Therapeutic investigations in primary sclerosing cholangitis. In: Huitbregtse K, ed. Endoscopic Biliary and Pancreatic Drainage. Stuttgart, FRG: Georg Thieme; 1988:78–85.
10. Cotton PB, Nickl N. Endoscopic and radiologic approaches to therapy in primary sclerosing cholangitis. Semin Liver Dis. 1991;11:40–8.
11. Craig PI, Hatfield RW. Endoscopic therapy in primary sclerosing cholangitis. Eur J Gastroenterol Hepatol. 1992;4:284–7.
12. Gaing AA, Geders JM, Cohen SA, Siegel JH. Endoscopic management of primary sclerosing cholangitis: review, and report of an open series. Am J Gastroenterol. 1993;88:2000–8.
13. Lee JG, Schutz SM, England RE, Leung JW, Cotton PB. Endoscopic therapy of sclerosing cholangitis. Hepatology. 1995;21:661–7.
14. van Milligen AWM, van Bracht J, Rauws EAJ *et al.* Endoscopic stent therapy for dominant extrahepatic bile duct strictures in primary sclerosing cholangitis. Gastrointest Endosc. 1996; 44:293–9.
15. Broome U, Olson R, Lööf L *et al.* Natural history and prognostic factors in 305 Swedish patients with primary sclerosing cholangitis. Gut. 1996;38:610–15.
16. Aadland E, Schrumpf E, Fausa O *et al.* Primary sclerosing cholangitis: long-term follow up study. Scand J Gastroenterol. 1987;22:655–64.
17. Helzberg JH, Petersen JM, Boyer JL. Improved survival with primary sclerosing cholangitis; a review of clinicopathologic features and comparison of symptomatic and asymptomatic patients. Gastroenterology. 1987;92:1869–75.
18. Lebovics E, Palmer M, Woo J *et al.* Outcome of primary sclerosing cholangitis. Arch Intern Med. 1987;147:729–31.
19. Herrmann R, Dooley J, Sherlock S, McIntyre N. Progression of asymptomatic primary sclerosing cholangitis. Abstract. J Hepatol. 1988;7:S39.
20. Farrant MJ, Hayllar KM, Wilkinson ML *et al.* Natural history and prognostic variables in primary sclerosing cholangitis. Gastroenterology. 1991;100:1710–17.
21. Wiesner RH, Grambsch PM, Dickson ER *et al.* Natural history, prognostic factors, and survival analysis. Hepatology. 1989;10:430–6.

11
Immunosuppressive therapy in primary sclerosing cholangitis

M. M. KAPLAN

Primary sclerosing cholangitis (PSC) is a chronic progressive liver disorder characterized by chronic fibrosing inflammation of both intra- and extrahepatic bile ducts, obliteration of bile ducts and the eventual development of biliary cirrhosis[1]. Until 1970, PSC was considered to be a medical curiosity. Fewer than 100 patients with PSC had been reported. However, the development of endoscopic cholangiography changed our perception of this disease. It is now recognized more frequently and, after chronic hepatitis C and alcoholic cirrhosis, is one of the common indications for liver transplantation. Approximately 4% of patients with inflammatory bowel disease (IBD) either have or will develop PSC. PSC can also occur in the absence of IBD[2].

The course of PSC is unpredictable but is usually progressive. It typically leads to cirrhosis, portal hypertension and the need for liver transplantation. The manifestations of disease may be clinically similar to those of other types of extrahepatic bile duct obstruction and PSC must be distinguished from gallstone disease, bile duct carcinoma, primary biliary cirrhosis and secondary biliary cirrhosis due to bile duct stricture. The disease may present in two forms: an acute form that is characterized by recurring episodes of fever, chills, right-upper-quadrant pain, jaundice and dark urine, and a more indolent form that is initially asymptomatic and recognized by abnormal liver function tests, typically elevated alkaline phosphatase. Patients who are asymptomatic and have normal serum bilirubin levels at diagnosis survive longer than symptomatic patients but still have shortened survival compared with a healthy age- and sex-matched population[3]. Median survival (that is, referral for liver transplantation) in asymptomatic patients is approximately 12 years.

IMMUNOSUPPRESSION AS TREATMENT FOR PCS

A variety of immunosuppressive, anti-inflammatory and antifibrotic agents have been used to treat PSC. However, no drug has been shown to improve its natural history. The evaluation of treatment has been limited by the unpredictable course of PSC and by the great variation in the severity of the disease at presentation. The course of PSC is indolent in most patients but may be rapidly progressive in some and associated with spontaneous exacerbations and remissions in others. Hence, even if a drug is effective, it will probably be years before its efficacy can be proven. Endoscopic approaches to treatment and the use of ursodeoxycholic acid in PSC are discussed elsewhere in this symposium. The experience with immunosuppressive, anti-inflammatory, and antifibrotic drugs will be reviewed here.

Corticosteroids and azathioprine

Despite anecdotal reports of improvement with glucocorticoids and azathioprine in patients with PSC[4,5], there is little enthusiasm for their use. Approximately 75% of patients with PSC have chronic IBD and were being treated with glucocorticoids and/or azathioprine or 6-mercaptopurine while PSC developed and progressed. Furthermore, combination treatment with colchicine and glucocorticoids is not effective[6]. Finally, glucocorticoids may accelerate the onset and progression of osteoporosis and increase spontaneous bone fractures. There is, however, one favourable report. In an uncontrolled trial, 10 patients with prefibrotic PSC had improvement in blood tests and liver histology. Four of these patients are well after 12 years and are still on low-dose prednisone (LaBrecque DR, personal communication).

D-Penicillamine

D-Penicillamine was evaluated in a double-blind prospective trial in 70 patients followed for 36 months[7]. D-Penicillamine produced the expected cupriuresis but had no beneficial effect on symptoms, biochemical tests, liver histology, disease progression or survival. In addition, 21% of the patients developed major side-effects from the drug. The toxicity and lack of efficacy have discouraged further use of D-penicillamine.

Cyclosporin

Cyclosporin was evaluated in a prospective double-blind trial in 34 patients followed for 24 months[8]. Twenty-two patients received cyclosporin and 12 placebo. Cyclosporin doses were adjusted to keep trough blood levels between 80 and 100 ng/ml (HPLC whole blood) and averaged 3.1 $mg\,kg^{-1}\,day^{-1}$. Thirty patients had repeat liver biopsies. After two years of treatment, cyclosporin had no beneficial effect on pruritus, fatigue, biochemical tests of liver function or survival free of liver transplantation. Nine of 10 patients on placebo showed histological progression of disease (90%) compared with 11 of 20 (55%) on cyclosporin. The authors concluded that cyclosporin was not effective in the treatment of PSC.

Colchicine

Eighty-four patients with PSC were randomized to receive either colchicine, 1 mg per day, or placebo, in a three-year double-blind study[9]. Liver biopsies were taken at baseline and at three years. Patients were evaluated every 6 months. Colchicine had no beneficial effect on symptoms, biochemical tests of liver function, liver histology or survival; it was clearly ineffective.

Methotrexate

Methotrexate has been evaluated at the New England Medical Center during the past 17 years, based on favourable experiences with 2 patients treated in 1979 and 1980. These 2 men had dramatic symptomatic, biochemical and histological responses while receiving methotrexate[10]. In an open-label study[11] of 10 patients, none of whom had clinically advanced disease, all patients had improvement in serum alkaline phosphatase while on oral methotrexate, approximately $0.25\,mg\,kg^{-1}\,week^{-1}$. Symptoms of right-upper-quadrant pain, fever, chills, itching and recurrent jaundice improved in the 6 patients who had these symptoms. Histology improved in 6 of 9 patients and was unchanged in 3. Patients with advanced disease, that is cirrhosis and portal hypertension, did not respond to methotrexate, ursodeoxycholic acid or the combination of these two, and the addition of antibiotics to these two drugs did not help in these patients with advanced disease. In a double-blind study, there was no therapeutic benefit for patients receiving methotrexate compared with those on placebo[12]. Twenty-four patients were randomized. Twelve received methotrexate, 15 mg/week and 12 placebo. Each patient was followed closely for 2 years or until he/she worsened clinically and was deemed a 'treatment failure'. The only statistically significant change was a decrease in the serum alkaline phosphatase in the patients receiving methotrexate. Just as many patients deteriorated clinically on methotrexate as on placebo. Half of the 24 patients in the study already had cirrhosis when enrolled, including 7 of the 12 patients receiving methotrexate. Patients with cirrhosis probably have medically irreversible PSC. Hence, there were only 5 patients on methotrexate who might have responded. One of those dropped out after one year because of a colectomy for exacerbation of ulcerative colitis. Of the 4 remaining patients, 3 patients appeared to improve. There was no toxicity from methotrexate. However, there is still no evidence that methotrexate by itself favourably affects the natural history of PSC.

Tacrolimus

Tacrolimus was evaluated in 10 patients who were followed for one year. After one year, the median serum bilirubin had fallen by 75%, the alkaline phosphatase by 70% and aminotransferases by 83%. The dose was that which kept trough levels of tacrolimus between 0.6 and 1.0 ng/ml[13]. No toxicity was reported. There were no data on liver histology or cholangiography. The short duration and uncontrolled nature of the study do not allow tacrolimus to be evaluated meaningfully as a treatment for PSC.

Suggestions

The negative results with both immunosuppressive therapy and ursodeoxycholic acid should prompt us to re-evaluate our approach to treatment and consider why there has been so little progress. The lack of effective drug therapy in PSC stands in contrast to other liver diseases, such as chronic hepatitis B and C, autoimmune chronic hepatitis and primary biliary cirrhosis, where there have been advances. There are at least three factors which contribute to our failure to find effective treatment for PSC. First is our poor understanding of its aetiology; second, our inability to diagnose the disease at its earliest stages, when it may be more amenable to treatment; and third, the lack of clinical trials utilizing combinations of different classes of drug, an approach which has proved effective in other complex diseases, such as AIDS and Hodgkin's disease.

Primary sclerosing cholangitis appears to be more complicated than other liver diseases and is most likely to be caused by multiple interacting pathogenetic factors. These include an immunologically impaired host, multiple bile duct strictures that impede bile flow, and chronic bile duct infection. The occurrence of multiple intrahepatic and extrahepatic bile duct strictures which obstruct bile flow makes effective antimicrobial therapy difficult if not impossible. Cholangiography identifies only strictures in large bile ducts and underestimates the severity of the problem. Biopsy findings suggest that many intrahepatic bile ducts, most too small to be visualized radiologically, are also obstructed.

The evidence that primary sclerosing cholangitis is an autoimmune disease is tentative. The familial occurrence, association with Class I and Class II haplotypes and abnormalities of immunoregulation have all been recently reviewed[1]. Most intriguing is the close association of primary sclerosing cholangitis with inflammatory bowel disease, another presumed autoimmune disease. The study of animal models suggests that inflammatory bowel disease may be caused by an interaction between normal intestinal bacteria and genetic abnormalities of immunoregulation and/or host defences, such as the lack of intestinal trefoil factor[14]. These abnormalities weaken host resistance and allow normal gut flora to become invasive[14,15]. Inflammatory bowel disease does not occur in the germ-free animal[15]. The pathogenesis of PSC may be similar; that is, it occurs in genetically susceptible hosts who have impaired defence mechanisms. Normal gut flora may then cause chronic bile duct infection. If this model is accurate, the best time to treat is early, before there are strictures that limit the efficacy of antibiotics. There are few data at this time to support the presence of chronic bile duct infection other than the observations that: (1) some patients with early-stage disease have recurrent episodes of chills and fever, (2) bacterial cholangitis is common in advanced disease, and (3) the incidence of infection is higher in patients with PSC after invasive procedures, such as endoscopic cholangiography and liver biopsy, than in other liver diseases. Bile, even in the normal host, is not sterile. An organ with multiple duct obstructions is therefore an ideal setting for chronic infection.

The second problem in developing new treatment strategies is our inability to diagnose PSC at its earliest stages. There is currently no biochemical, serological or commonly occurring histological abnormality that allows early diagnosis. The cholestatic pattern of blood tests is non-specific. Perinuclear antineutrophil cytoplasmic antibody, a candidate serological test, is insensitive and non-specific[16]. The pathognomonic onionskin lesion is rarely seen on percutaneous biopsy. The cholangiographic changes used to diagnose primary sclerosing cholangitis reflect diffuse bile duct scarring. Their presence suggests that the disease is already advanced and medically irreversible. The current biochemical and histological criteria for staging this disease are insensitive and misclassify as early disease many patients whose bile duct scarring may already be far advanced. We need criteria that do not require cholangiographic evidence of structuring. Once stricturing occurs, there is no drug currently available that can reverse it. The goal is to control inflammation and/or infection and prevent scarring.

Based on the above considerations, I suggest that progress will only be made when it is possible to diagnose PSC at an early stage, before there are tight strictures that are obvious on cholangiography, and when combination therapy is used as treatment. Such therapy should include antibiotics, ursodeoxycholic acid and immunosuppressive agents.

References

1. Lee YM, Kaplan MM. Primary sclerosing cholangitis. N Engl J Med. 1995;332:924–33.
2. Lindor K, Wiesner R, LaRusso N. Recent advances in the management of primary sclerosing cholangitis. Semin Liver Dis. 1987;7:322–7.
3. Wiesner RH, Grambsch PM, Dickson ER *et al.* Primary sclerosing cholangitis: natural history, prognostic factors and survival analysis. Hepatology. 1989;10:430–6.
4. Myers RN, Cooper JH, Padis N. Primary sclerosing cholangitis: complete gross and histologic reversal after long-term steroid therapy. Am J Gastroenterol. 1970;53:527–38.
5. Wagner A. Azathioprine treatment in primary sclerosing cholangitis. Lancet. 1971;2:663–4.
6. Lindor KD, Wiesner RH, Colwell LJ, Steiner B, Beaver S, LaRusso NF. The combination of prednisone and colchicine in patients with primary sclerosing cholangitis. Am J Gastroenterol. 1991; 86:57–61.
7. LaRusso NF, Wiesner RH, Ludwig J, MacCarty RL, Beaver SJ, Zinsmeister AR. Prospective trial of penicillamine in primary sclerosing cholangitis. Gastroenterology. 1988;95:1036–42.
8. Wiesner R, Steiner B, LaRusso N, Lindor K, Baldus W. A controlled clinical trial evaluating cyclosporin in the treatment of primary sclerosing cholangitis. Hepatology. 1991;14:63A.
9. Olsson R, Broome U, Danielsson A *et al.* Colchicine treatment of primary sclerosing cholangitis. Gastroenterology. 1995;108:1199–203.
10. Kaplan MM, Arora S, Pincus SH. Primary sclerosing cholangitis and low dose oral pulse methotrexate. Ann Intern Med. 1987;106:231–5.
11. Knox TA, Kaplan MM. Treatment of primary sclerosing cholangitis with oral methotrexate. Am J Gastroenterol. 1991;86:546–52.
12. Knox TA, Kaplan MM. A double-blind controlled trial of oral-pulse methotrexate therapy in the treatment of primary sclerosing cholangitis [see comments]. Gastroenterology. 1994;106:494–9.
13. Van Thiel DH, Carroll P, Abu-Elmagd K *et al.* Tacrolimus (FK 506), a treatment for primary sclerosing cholangitis: results of an open-label preliminary trial. Am J Gastroenterol. 1995;90: 455–9.
14. Mashimo H, Wu D, Podolsky D, Fishman M. Impaired defense of intestinal mucosa in mice lacking intestinal trefoil factor. Science. 1996;274:262–5.
15. Elson C, Sartor R, Tennyson G, Riddell R. Experimental models of inflammatory bowel disease. Gastroenterology. 1995;109:1344–67.
16. Duerr DH, Targan SR, Landers CJ *et al.* Neutrophil cytoplasmic antibodies: a link between primary sclerosing cholangitis and ulcerative colitis. Gastroenterology. 1991;100:1385–91.

12
Endoscopic treatment of primary sclerosing cholangitis

S. WAGNER, P. N. MEIER and M. P. MANNS

INTRODUCTION

Primary sclerosing cholangitis (PSC) is a chronic cholestatic liver disease of unknown aetiology. It is characterized by inflammation, destruction, and fibrosis of intrahepatic and extrahepatic bile ducts[1,2]. The natural history of PSC is characterized by remissions and exacerbations, frequently terminating in cirrhosis and liver failure which may require liver transplantation[3–6]. No currently accepted form of therapy exists for this disease, and preliminary promising results with ursodeoxycholic acid could not be confirmed in a recent placebo-controlled study[7–12]. Various surgical strategies have been unsuccessful in preventing recurrent attacks of cholangitis[13–16]. Recent studies employing endoscopic methods show beneficial effects of that therapy in selected patients with dominant bile duct strictures[17–21]. Therefore, the aim of this chapter is to discuss the indications, methods, and results of endoscopic treatment in PSC patients.

ROLE OF ENDOSCOPIC RETROGRADE CHOLANGIOPANCREATOGRAPHY (ERCP) IN THE MANAGEMENT OF PSC

ERCP plays a central role in the management of PSC. Cholangiography is not only the gold standard for diagnosis of PSC but it also gives some information on the prognosis of the disease. High-grade strictures and diffuse strictures of the intrahepatic ducts have been identified as indicators of poor prognosis[22]. ERCP is also of importance in the evaluation and management of complications of PSC. In the follow-up of PSC patients, diagnostic cholangiography is indicated if recurrent cholangitis develops, or if there is a rapid deterioration of liver function. Therapeutic endoscopic measures are required if there are bile duct stones or dominant strictures of the major bile ducts.

ENDOSCOPIC TREATMENT MODALITIES IN PSC PATIENTS

Table 1 summarizes the different endoscopic treatment modalities in PSC patients. Endoscopic sphincterotomy of the papilla of Vater is rarely used alone as a single treatment modality, but is most commonly performed to facilitate further endoscopic manoeuvres. There are few anecdotal reports claiming that the sphincterotomy alone improves biliary drainage[20]. For the reopening of dominant bile duct stenoses endoscopic dilation therapy is especially suited. There are two different dilation tools: angioplasty-type balloon catheters and coaxial dilators. The balloon catheters allow application of high pressure (10 bar) at a defined outer diameter (5–10 mm). The coaxial dilators are helpful in very tight strictures where a balloon catheter cannot be passed. After dilating a stricture with coaxial dilators, a balloon catheter can be introduced in the stricture, and maximal dilation of the stricture subsequently is accomplished. For long-lasting reopening of biliary strictures by dilation therapy multiple treatment sessions are necessary[21,23]. Endoscopic placement of endoprostheses is an alternative method for management of biliary strictures. Stenting provides immediate biliary drainage, especially in high-grade strictures. The main problem of endoprostheses is the recurrent occlusion of the stents associated with bacterial cholangitis. Therefore stents should be removed or changed after 3 months. Another endoscopic treatment modality in PSC is biliary lavage by nasobiliary perfusion. This allows removal of biliary exudate and debris, and is usually combined with dilation therapy.

INDICATION AND METHOD OF ENDOSCOPIC TREATMENT OF BILIARY STRICTURES

An endoscopic treatment of biliary stenoses in PSC is indicated if focal dominant strictures of the extrahepatic bile duct, including the right and left hepatic duct, are suspected, and if there is evidence of cholestasis. The condition implies that only a minority of PSC patients will be suited for endoscopic therapy,

Table 1 Endoscopic treatment modalities in PSC patients: overview and features

Endoscopic sphincterotomy of the papilla
Only anecdotal reports to suggest a supportive effect on biliary drainage
Rarely used as a single treatment modality
Endoscopic dilation of biliary strictures
Dilation material: (a) angioplasty-type, high-pressure balloon catheters; (b) co-axial dilators
Multiple interventions necessary for long-lasting reopening of strictures
Endoscopic placement of endoprostheses
Immediate and effective therapy for high-grade strictures
Problem of recurrent stent occlusion and bacterial cholangitis
Stents have to be removed/changed after 3 months
Biliary lavage
Removal of inflammation-associated exudate, sludge, debris
Frequently combined with other treatment modalities

representing about 20–30% of PSC patients. Diffuse intrahepatic strictures cannot be treated endoscopically.

Table 2 summarizes the treatment strategy of the Medizinische Hochschule Hannover for management of biliary strictures in PSC patients[21]. All patients receive antibiotic prophylaxis. If dominant strictures are identified and endoscopic therapy is planned we routinely perform a sphincterotomy to facilitate insertion of the balloon catheter and to separate the bile duct orifice from the pancreas, thereby minimizing the risk of complicating pancreatitis. A guidewire is placed into the stenotic bile duct and an angioplasty catheter (Olbert catheter, 4.8–7.8 F, balloon diameter 5–10 mm, pressure 10 bar, Meadox Surgimed A/S, Ratingen, Germany) is advanced through the stricture under fluoroscopic control. Dilation is performed by serial inflations (1 min) of the balloon with physiological saline (supplemented with contrast medium) up to a maximum pressure of 10 bar. If multiple dominant strictures are present, each of them may be treated during one session. Subsequently, a nasobiliary catheter is inserted through the most proximal dominant stricture into an intrahepatic portion of the biliary system for irrigation (500–1000 ml/day). After irrigating the biliary tree for 1 week, balloon dilation is repeated. Our preference is to place an endoprosthesis because of frequent stent occlusion and the development of complicated bacterial cholangitis. However, in a case of unsuccessful reopening of strictures by balloon dilation, stent placement is indicated. All patients continue treatment with ursodeoxycholic acid (UDCA).

RESULTS OF ENDOSCOPIC TREATMENT OF BILIARY STRICTURES

In an ongoing prospective series at the Medizinische Hochschule Hannover, 24 symptomatic PSC patients (14 men, 10 women, mean age 38 ± 11 years) with dominant strictures were allocated to endoscopic treatment as outlined above. A total of 51 major strictures were detected in this group. Satisfactory reopening of the strictures was achieved in 44 of 51 strictures. On the average 3.5 sessions (range 2–10) of dilating therapy were necessary to obtain a sustained reopening of biliary strictures. The mean follow-up period for the total group of patients was 26 months (range 6–65 months). Eighteen of 24 PSC patients showed a long-lasting improvement following endoscopic therapy as assessed by clinical,

Table 2 Endoscopic therapy of biliary strictures in PSC: procedure and follow-up

Antibiotic prophylaxis (ciprofloxacin or mezlocillin)
Endoscopic sphincterotomy of the papilla
Dilation with angioplasty-type balloon catheter under fluoroscopic guidance
6–10 mm outer diameter
inflation with contrast medium diluted with saline, at a pressure of 10 bar
procedure repeated until complete reopening of the stricture
Nasobiliary catheter perfusion (normal saline 500–1000 ml/day) for 1 week
Repeat balloon dilation after 1 week
Cholangiographic follow-up at 3–12 month intervals; repeat dilation if necessary
Stent placement only if dilation treatment is unsuccessful
Continuation of UDCA treatment

laboratory and cholangiographic criteria. Four patients underwent liver transplantation because of deteriorating liver function. Two patients showed only a transient improvement.

There were only minor procedure-related side-effects. One patient experienced haemorrhage after endoscopic sphincterotomy which could be controlled without surgical intervention. Six episodes of pancreatitis were noted, which were managed by conservative routine measures. Episodes of cholangitis were observed in three patients, which were treated with antibiotics and repeat balloon dilations.

Figure 1 illustrates the effect of dilation therapy on laboratory data and stricture scores obtained in a recent pilot study[21]. There was a significant improve-

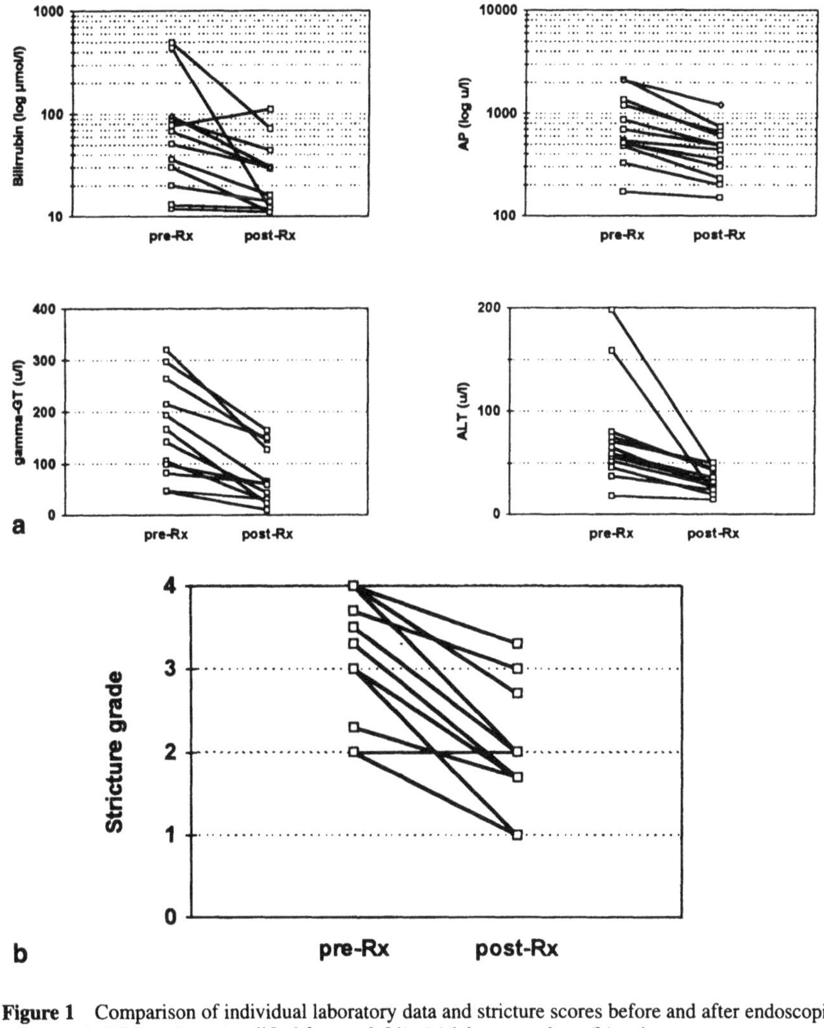

Figure 1 Comparison of individual laboratory data and stricture scores before and after endoscopic treatment in PSC patients (modified from ref. 21): (**a**) laboratory data, (**b**) stricture scores

ment of both the laboratory data and stricture scores in the majority of the patients.

Our results are in good agreement with previous reports employing different endoscopic treatment modalities in PSC patients (Table 3)[19,20,23-25]. In these trials follow-up varied between 24 and 52 months; overall about 60–80% showed an improvement of clinical, cholangiographic, and laboratory data. Unfortunately, controlled trials have not been performed up to now. Nonetheless, it may be concluded from current data that endoscopic treatment is effective and safe in selected patients with dominant strictures of the major bile ducts.

CONCLUSION

PSC is an increasingly recognized chronic cholestatic liver disease of unknown cause which is characterized by a slow but relentless progress leading to cirrhosis and liver failure. No specific treatment for PSC currently exists, although ursodiol has some beneficial effects. Liver transplantation is the treatment of choice for patients with advanced liver disease. Endoscopic treatment is indicated in symptomatic patients with dominant strictures of the major bile ducts. Repeated angioplasty-type balloon dilation and nasobiliary catheter perfusion are the treatment of choice for biliary stenoses. Endoscopic placement of endoprostheses is an alternative approach, but a major disadvantage of this method is the recurrent occlusion of the stents complicated by bacterial cholangitis.

Table 3 Endoscopic therapy of PSC: review of the literature

Stiehl *et al.*[23]	
Prospective study	$n=23$
Procedure	Balloon dilation and UDCA therapy
Follow-up	45 months
Outcome	*Improved survival compared to predicted rates*
van Milligen de Wit *et al.*[25]	
Retrospective study	$n=25$
Procedure	Stent therapy
Follow-up	29 months
Asymptomatic after treatment	*57%*
Lee *et al.*[24]	
Retrospective study	$n=53$
Procedure	dilation, stenting, nasobiliary tube
Follow-up	31 months
Overall improvement	*77%*
Gaing *et al.*[20]	
Retrospective study	$n=42$
Procedure	Dilation, stenting, nasobiliary perfusion
Follow-up	52 months
Biochemical improvement	*70%*
Johnson *et al.*[19]	
Retrospective study	$n=35$
Procedure	Dilation (stenting)
Follow-up	24 months
Overall improvement	*85%*

Endoscopic therapy results in a sustained reopening of biliary strictures which leads to an improvement of clinical, cholangiographic, and biochemical findings in the majority of patients. Thus, endoscopic therapy is an effective, safe, and well-tolerated measure for selected PSC patients with dominant strictures of the major bile ducts.

References

1. Lee YM, Kaplan MM. Primary sclerosing cholangitis. N. Engl J Med. 1995;332:924–33.
2. Wiener RH, Grambsch PM, Dickson ER *et al.* Primary sclerosing cholangitis: natural history, prognostic factors and survival analysis. Hepatology. 1989;10:430–6.
3. Dickson ER, Murtaugh PA, Wiesner RH *et al.* Primary sclerosing cholangitis: refinement and validation of survival models. Gastroenterology. 1992;103:1893–901.
4. Farrant JM, Hayllar KM, Wilkinson ML *et al.* Natural history and prognostic variables in primary sclerosing cholangitis. Gastroenterology. 1991;100:1710–17.
5. Kilpe VE, Krakauer H, Wren RE. An analysis of liver transplant experience from 37 transplant centers as reported to Medicare. Transplantation. 1993;56:554–61.
6. Abu Elmagd KM, Malinchoc M, Dickson ER *et al.* Efficacy of hepatic transplantation in patients with primary sclerosing cholangitis. Surg Gynecol Obstet. 1993;177:335–44.
7. Kaplan MM. Medical approaches to primary sclerosing cholangitis. Semin Liver Dis. 1991;11: 56–63.
8. O'Brien CB, Senior JR, Arora Mirchandani R, Batta AK, Salen G. Ursodeoxycholic acid for the treatment of primary sclerosing cholangitis: a 30-month pilot study. Hepatology. 1991;14: 838–47.
9. Beuers U, Spengler U, Kruis W. *et al.* Ursodeoxycholic acid for treatment of primary sclerosing cholangitis: a placebo-controlled trial. Hepatology. 1992;16:707–14.
10. Lebovics E, Salama M, Elhosseiny A, Rosenthal WS. Resolution of radiographic abnormalities with ursodeoxycholic acid therapy of primary sclerosing cholangitis. Gastroenterology. 1992; 102:2143–7.
11. Gross JB, Jr. Promises, promises: ursodeoxycholic acid for primary sclerosing cholangitis. Gastroenterology. 1993;104:941–3.
12. Lindor KD. Ursodiol for primary sclerosing cholangitis. Mayo Primary Sclerosing Cholangitis-Ursodeoxycholic Acid Study Group. N Engl J Med. 1997;336:691–5.
13. Pitt HA, Thompson HH, Tompkins RK, Longmire WP. Primary sclerosing cholangitis: results of an aggressive approach. Ann Surg. 1982;196:259–68.
14. Thompson JS, Wood RP, Burnett DA, Shaw BW, Rikkers LF. The role of non-transplant procedures for sclerosing cholangitis. Am J Surg. 1988;150:506–8.
15. Lillemoe KD, Cameron JL. Surgical approaches to primary sclerosing cholangitis. Semin Liver Dis. 1991;11:49–55.
16. Ismail T, Angrisani L, Powell JE *et al.* Primary sclerosing cholangitis: surgical options, prognostic variables and outcome. Br J Surg. 1991;78:564–7.
17. Cotton PB, Nickl N. Endoscopic and radiologic approaches to therapy in primary sclerosing cholangitis. Semin Liver Dis. 1991;11:40–8.
18. Lombard M, Farrant M, Karani J, Westaby D, Williams R. Improving biliary-enteric drainage in primary sclerosing cholangitis: experience with endoscopic methods. Gut 1991;32:1364–8.
19. Johnson GK, Geenen JE, Venu RP, Schmalz MJ, Hogan WJ. Endoscopic treatment of biliary tract strictures in sclerosing cholangitis: a larger series and recommendations for treatment. Gastrointest Endosc. 1991;37:38–43.
20. Gaing AA, Geders JM, Cohen SA, Siegel JH. Endoscopic management of primary sclerosing cholangitis: review, and report of an open series. Am J Gastroenterol. 1993;88:2000–8.
21. Wagner S, Gebel M, Meier P *et al.* Endoscopic management of biliary tract strictures in primary sclerosing cholangitis. Endoscopy. 1996;28:546–51.
22. Craig DA, MacCarty RL, Wiesner RH, Grambsch PM, LaRusso NF. Primary sclerosing cholangitis: value of cholangiography in determining the prognosis. Am J Roentgenol. 1991;157: 959–64.
23. Stiehl A, Rudolph G, Sauer P *et al.* Efficacy of ursodeoxycholic acid treatment and endoscopic

dilation of major duct stenoses in primary sclerosing cholangitis. An 8-year prospective study. J Hepatol. 1997;26:560–6.
24. Lee JG, Schutz SM, England RE, Leung JW, Cotton PB. Endoscopic therapy of sclerosing cholangitis. Hepatology. 1995;21:661–7.
25. van Milligen de Wit AW, van Bracht J, Rauws EA, Jones EA, Tytgat GN, Huibregtse K. Endoscopic stent therapy for dominant extrahepatic bile duct strictures in primary sclerosing cholangitis. Gastrointest Endosc. 1996;44:293–9.

13
Treatment of complications of primary sclerosing cholangitis

C. IJ. PONSIOEN and K. HUIBREGTSE

INTRODUCTION

Primary sclerosing cholangitis (PSC) is a chronic progressive cholestatic liver disease of unknown origin. It is characterized by fibro-obliterative inflammation of the entire biliary tree.

The estimated median survival or time to liver transplantation is about 12 years[1-3]. During the course of the disease, several complications can be encountered: (1) cholelithiasis, (2) suppurative cholangitis, (3) symptomatic dominant strictures, and (4) cholangiocarcinoma. These complications will be discussed below.

CHOLELITHIASIS

By convention, a diagnosis of PSC used to be excluded when cholelithiasis was present (Figure 1). However, Pokorny *et al.*, in a comparative study, found that patients with sclerosing cholangitis and biliary tract calculi were in no sense different from PSC patients who satisfied this exclusion criterion[4]. Biliary tract calculi seem to be a part of the spectrum of PSC, and in fact gallstones are found in 25–33% of these patients[5,6]. Not infrequently, the diagnosis of PSC is made by endoscopic retrograde cholangiopancreatography (ERCP) for presumed symptomatic gallstone disease (Figure 2).

Biliary stasis is the presumptive pathogenetic mechanism by which the increased tendency for stone formation is explained. Recurrent ascending cholangitis, promoted by impaired bile flow, can add to gallstone formation, especially brown pigment stones[7].

Bacteria are present in the biliary tract in up to 80% of patients with gallstones. PSC patients with choledocholitiasis are therefore more prone to recurrent suppurative cholangitis. Removal of gallstones in PSC patients is therefore considered essential to prevent cholangitis. Likewise, when cholecystolithiasis is present, elective cholecystectomy is usually thought to be indicated.

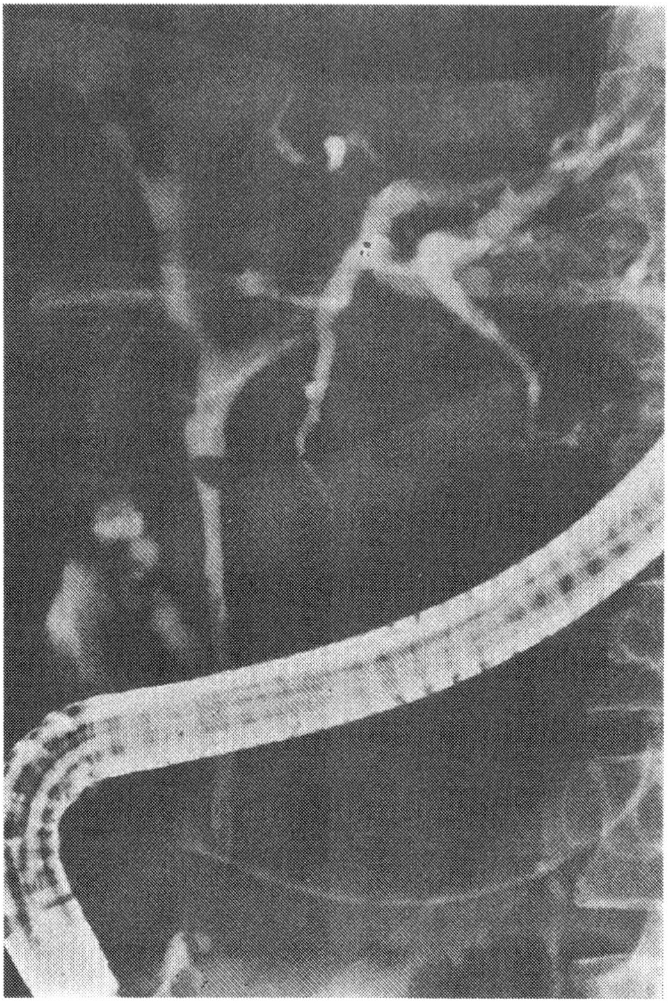

Figure 1 Gallstone in the common hepatic duct of a patient with PSC

SUPPURATIVE CHOLANGITIS

A well-known complication of PSC is suppurative cholangitis. This can occur either spontaneously or procedure related. The incidence of spontaneous cholangitis is not clearly established, but almost all patients sometimes experience episodes of chills, fever, pain and dark urine during the course of the disease. These complaints can be of short duration, but, when they do not rapidly subside, the patient should be treated with antibiotics and, if possible, a drainage procedure should be carried out.

The preferred antibiotics should cover the spectrum of expected causative micro-organisms and be tailored to the results of blood and/or bile cultures. The

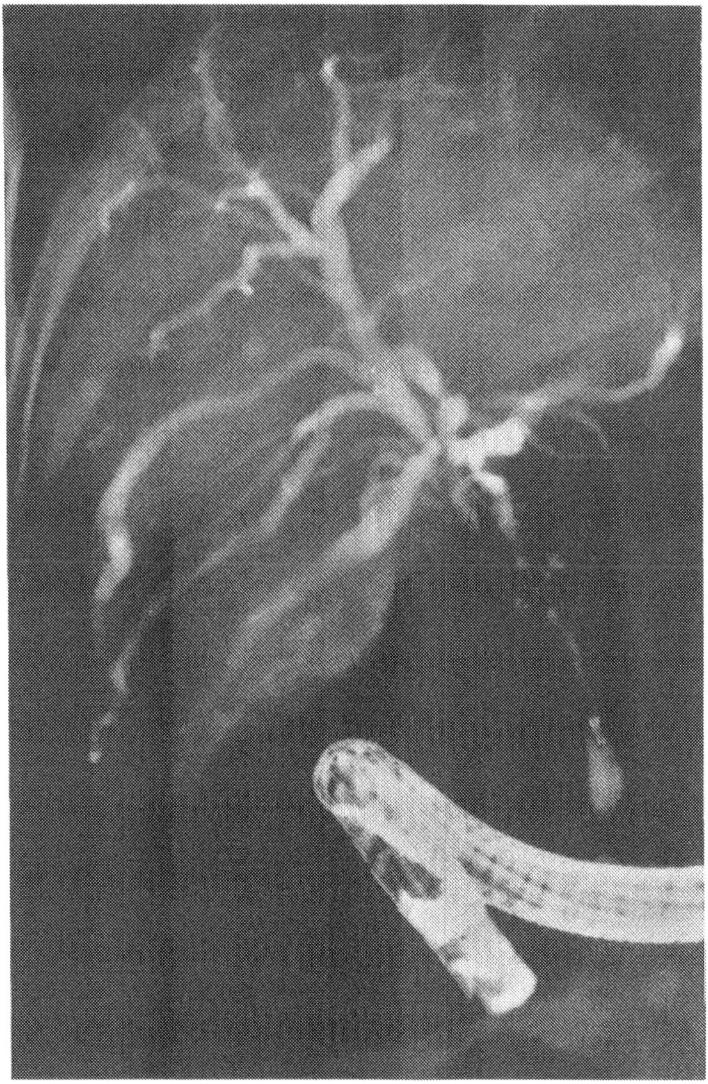

Figure 2 Cholangiogram showing the typical features of PSC: long stricture of the extrahepatic bile duct with saccular outpouchings; intrahepatic irregularities of the biliary system

most common organisms found in compromised biliary tracts are Gram-negative bacteria, in particular *Escherichia coli* and *Klebsiella* spp. To a lesser extent, other Gram-negative rods and *Enterococcus faecalis* can be found. Not infrequently, more than one species is cultured[8–11].

Amoxicillin and gentamicin are mostly used for in-patients until the results of blood and bile cultures are available. For out-patients, ciprofloxacin orally is a good alternative. This is the only antibiotic agent with a non-impaired biliary excretion in case of biliary obstruction[12]. The drainage procedure of choice nowadays is via ERCP. Common bile duct stones can be removed endoscopically, strictures can be treated by stents or balloon dilatation and nasobiliary drains can be inserted to clean the bile ducts of sludge and debris (Figures 3 and 4).

SYMPTOMATIC DOMINANT STRICTURES

When a tight stricture occurs in the common bile duct or the main branches to the left and right lobe, it is called a dominant stricture. The exact prevalence of these strictures is not known, but has been estimated to be around 10% in a large group of patients with PSC[13]. Patients who develop a dominant stricture com-

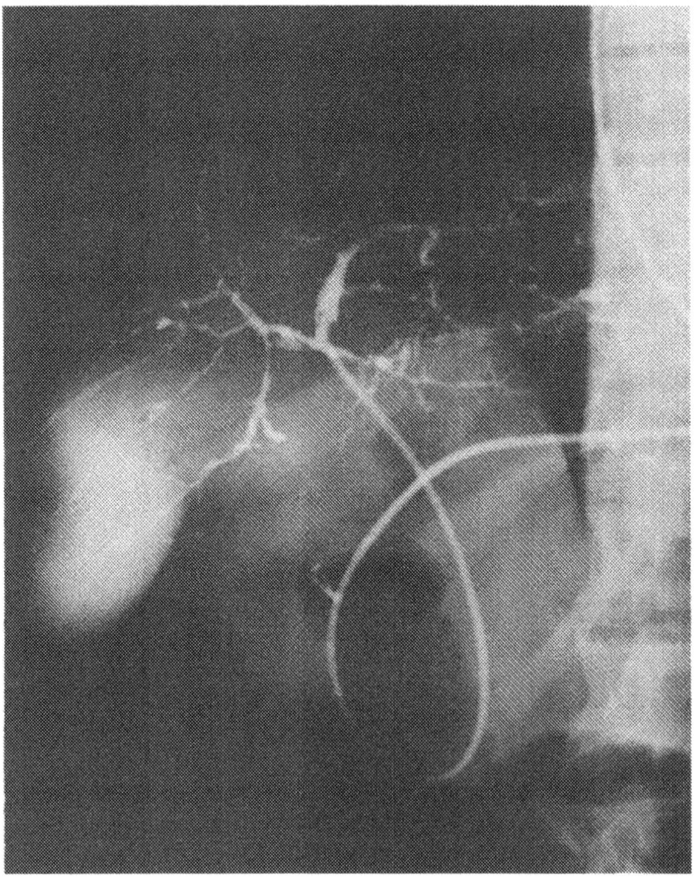

Figure 3 Nasobiliary drain through the extrahepatic bile duct stricture in a severely diseased intrahepatic biliary system to clean the bile ducts by flushing

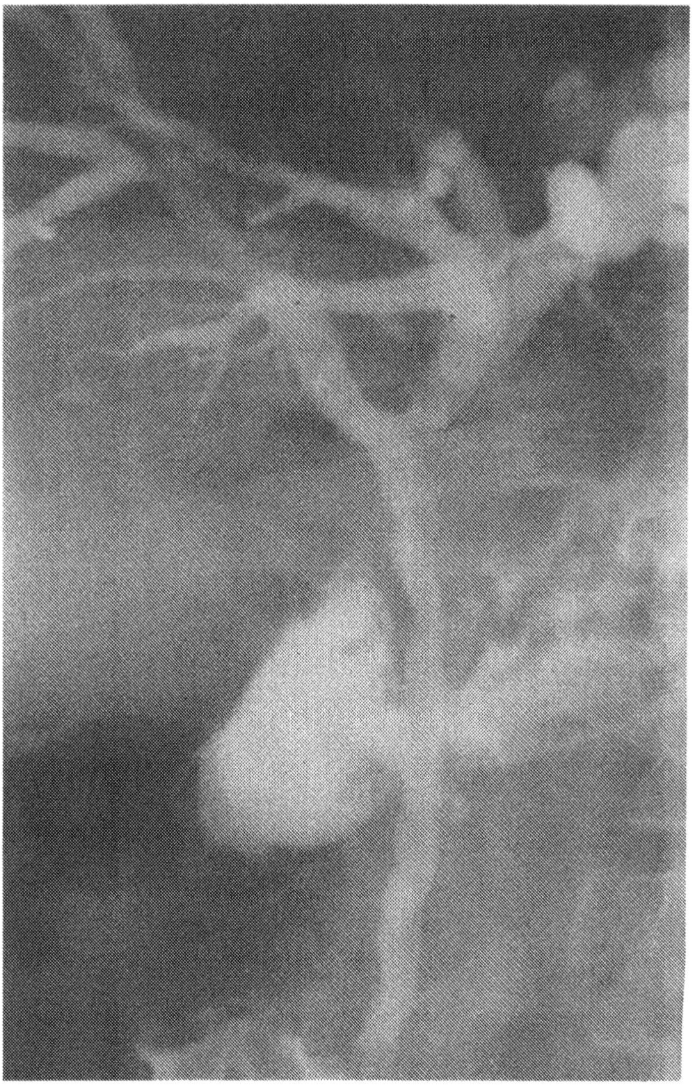

Figure 4 Much improved biliary system (see Figure 1) after 33(!) ERCPs for stone removal, nasobiliary drainage, and stricture dilatation with balloons and stents

monly present with symptoms of progressive cholestasis, i.e. jaundice, pruritus or cholangitis.

In the management of symptomatic dominant strictures, several approaches have been employed.

Percutaneous transhepatic cholangiography with balloon dilatation and temporary stenting has been reported to improve clinical, laboratory and radiological parameters[14]. However, it can be a technically difficult procedure, particularly because, frequently, the intrahepatic bile ducts are not conveniently dilated.

With the advent of endoscopic retrograde cholangiography, several series have been published, employing bougienage, balloon dilatation and/or placement of an endoprosthesis[15–18].

Balloon dilatation of PSC-related dominant strictures was first described in 1983[19]. Since then, several authors have reported favourable results of endoscopic dilatation[15,16].

Recurrent stricture formation is a well-recognized problem, although the precise incidence has not been documented. Some investigators prefer to insert an endoprosthesis afterwards, which is then left in place for several months[17].

It is not known how long an endoprosthesis should ideally be left *in situ* to achieve optimal dilatation effect with a minimum of stent-related complications, such as stent clogging or suppurative cholangitis[18] (Figure 5).

Because of the problem of stent clogging, we performed a trial in which the efficacy of short-term stent placement for symptomatic dominant strictures in PSC patients was evaluated[20].

Sixteen patients received one or two stents for cholangitis, jaundice, or progressive cholestasis. The mean duration of stent placement was 9 days (range 7–23). The median follow-up was 19 months (range 7–27 months). The results so far show that a 1-week stent placement is effective and comparable to the previously mentioned studies. No stent-related complications were seen. We have now adopted this treatment as the standard therapy for dominant strictures (Figure 6).

After placement of a polyethylene endoprosthesis, the patients are observed in hospital for 24 h to monitor complications, such as suppurative cholangitis,

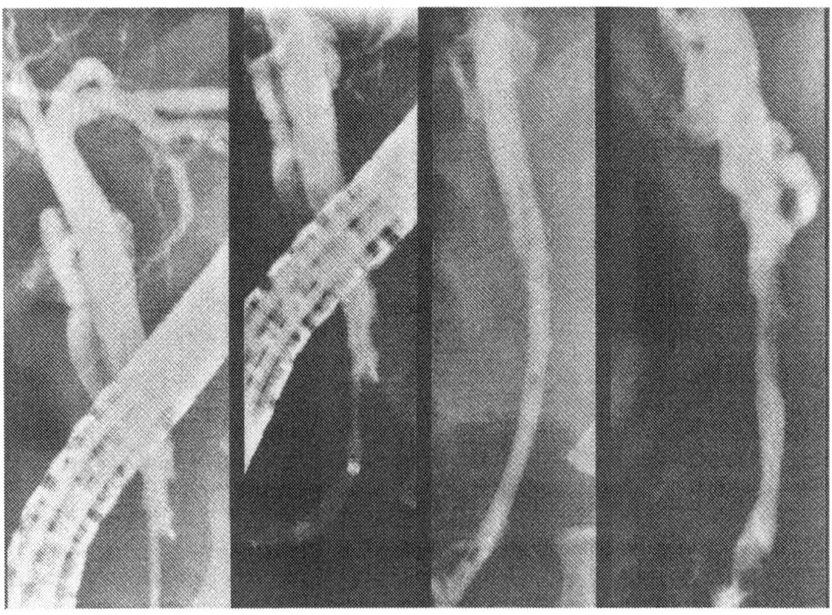

Figure 5 Dominant distal common bile stricture (left). Biliary stent for dilatation (centre). Dilated stricture (right)

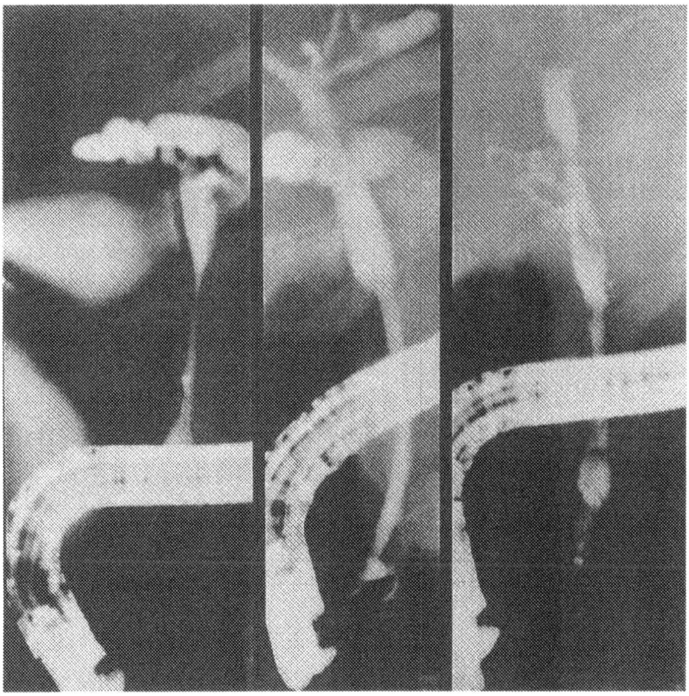

Figure 6 Smooth bile duct stricture (left). Stent inserted through stricture (middle). Result after 1 week's stenting (right)

pancreatitis and, especially when the common bile duct is very narrow at the level of the insertion of the cystic duct, hydrops of the gallbladder.

CHOLANGIOCARCINOMA

A very dismal complication of PSC is the development of cholangiocarcinoma. In the 3 larger studies mentioned earlier, this occurred in 6–8% of patients. It is possible that this may be an underestimate of the true incidence, since not all patients who die from liver failure are autopsied. Also, longstanding duration of liver disease is not a prerequisite for the development of cholangiocarcinoma[21]. Clinically as well as cholangiographically, cholangiocarcinoma can have a presentation similar to that of dominant stricture.

Detection of cholangiocarcinoma prior to OLT is important, because approximately 70% of patients with this complication, even when found incidentally in the resected liver, die within 1 year after OLT[3,21,22]. Abu-Elmagd *et al.* found, in their group of 169 transplanted PSC patients, 18 cholangiocarcinomas (10.6%), for which the 5-year survival rate was 26.7%[23].

The diagnosis of cholangiocarcinoma can be made by brush cytology of suspicious strictures. The reliability of brush cytology is, however, questionable.

In our experience, false negative and, especially after stenting, false positive results are possible. Noteworthy is the study from Rabinovitz *et al.* who claim that the sensitivity can be enhanced by repeated brushings up to 3 times[24]. In the presence of thin-walled sacculations, we consider biopsy too hazardous because of the risk of perforation.

The only therapy at present for cholangiocarcinoma in PSC is orthotopic liver transplantation (OLT). However, since the chance of curation is virtually nil, PSC patients with cholangiocarcinoma are excluded from OLT in most centres.

Recently, p53 protein over-expression was found in most cholangiocarcinoma specimens of PSC patients but not in liver tissue of PSC patients without cholangiocarcinoma[25]. K-ras oncogene mutations have also been demonstrated in cholangiocarcinoma[26]. Perhaps, along these lines, it will be possible in the future to detect cholangiocarcinoma in an earlier stage when a curative resection is still possible.

References

1. Broomé U, Olsson R, Loof L *et al.* Natural history and prognostic factors in 305 Swedish patients with primary sclerosing cholangitis. Gut. 1996;38:610–15.
2. Wiesner RH, Grambsch PM *et al.* Primary sclerosing cholangitis: natural history, prognostic factors and survival analysis. Hepatology. 1989;10:430–6.
3. Farrant M, Williams R. Natural history and prognosis in primary sclerosing cholangitis. Eur J Gastroenterol Hepatol. 1992;4:272–5.
4. Pokorny CS, McCaughan GW, Gallagher ND *et al.* Sclerosing cholangitis and biliary tract calculi–primary or secondary? Gut. 1992;33:1376–80.
5. Kaw M, Silverman WB, Rabinovitz M *et al.* Biliary tract calculi in primary sclerosing cholangitis. Am J Gastroenterol. 1995;90:72–5.
6. Wiesner RH, Ludwig J, LaRusso NF *et al.* Diagnosis and treatment of primary sclerosing cholangitis. Semin Liver Dis. 1985;5:241–53.
7. Cetta FM. Bile infection documented as the initial event in the pathogenesis of brown pigment stones. Hepatology. 1986;6:482–9.
8. Dowidar N, Kolmos HJ, Lyon H *et al.* Clogging of biliary endoprosthesis. A morphologic and bacteriologic study. Scand J Gastroenterol. 1991;26:1137–44.
9. Coene PPLO. Endoscopic Biliary Stenting. Thesis, Department of Gastroenterology and Hepatology. Amsterdam: University of Amsterdam; 1990:205.
10. Pitt HA, Postier RG, Cameron JL. Biliary bacteria. Significance and alterations after antibiotic therapy. Arch Surg. 1982;117:445–9.
11. Maluenda F, Csendes A, Burdiles P *et al.* Bacteriological study of choledochal bile in patients with common bile duct stones, with or without suppurative cholangitis. Hepatogastroenterology. 1989;36:132–5.
12. Hazel van den SJ. Antibiotics in the Prevention of Cholangitis. Thesis, Department of Gastroenterology and Hepatology. Amsterdam: University of Amsterdam; 1996:111.
13. MacCarty RL, LaRusso NF, Wiesner RH *et al.* Primary sclerosing cholangitis: findings on cholangiography and pancreaticography. Radiology. 1983;149:39–44.
14. May GR, Bender CE, LaRusso NR *et al.* Nonoperative dilatation of dominant strictures in primary sclerosing cholangitis. Am J Radiol. 1985;145:1061–4.
15. Johnson GK, Geenen JE, Venu RP *et al.* Endoscopic treatment of biliary tract strictures in sclerosing cholangitis: a larger series and recommendations for treatment. Gastrointest Endosc. 1991;37:38–43.
16. Lee JG, Schutz SM, Leung JW *et al.* Endoscopic therapy of sclerosing cholangitis. Hepatology. 1995;21:661–7.
17. Gaing AA, Geders JM, Cohen SA *et al.* Endoscopic management of primary sclerosing cholangitis: review, and report of an open series [Review]. Am J Gastroenterol. 1993;88:2000–8.
18. Milligen de Wit van AWM, Bracht v J, Rauws EAJ *et al.* Endoscopic stent therapy for dominant

extrahepatic bile duct strictures in primary sclerosing cholangitis. Gastrointest Endosc. 1996; 44:293–9.
19. Siegel JH, Guelrud M. Endoscopic cholangiopancreatoplasty: Hydrostatic balloon dilation in the bile duct and the pancreas. Gastrointest Endosc. 1983;29:99–103.
20. Milligen de Wit van M, Bracht van J, Rauws EAJ *et al.* Short-term endoscopic stent therapy for dominant extrahepatic bile duct strictures in primary sclerosing cholangitis. Neth J Med. 1995;47:A22.
21. Marsh JW, Iwatsuki S, Makowka L *et al.* Orthotopic liver transplantation for primary sclerosing cholangitis. Ann Surg. 1988;207:21–5.
22. Nashan B, Schlitt HJ, Tusch G *et al.* Biliary malignancies in primary sclerosing cholangitis: timing for liver transplantation. Hepatology. 1996;23:1105–11.
23. Abu-Elmagd KM, Selby R, Iwatsuki S *et al.* Cholangiocarcinoma and sclerosing cholangitis: clinical characteristics and effect on survival after liver transplantation. Transplant Proc. 1993; 25:1124–5.
24. Rabinovitz M, Zajko AB, Hassanein T *et al.* Diagnostic value of brush cytology in the diagnosis of bile duct carcinoma: a study of 65 patients with bile duct strictures. Hepatology. 1990; 12:747–52.
25. Rizzi PM, Ryder SD, Portmann B *et al.* p53 Protein over expression in cholangiocarcinoma arising in primary sclerosing cholangitis. Gut. 1996;38:265–8.
26. Levi S, Urbano-Ispizua A, Gill R *et al.* Multiple K-ras codon 12 mutations in cholangiocarcinomas demonstrated with a sensitive polymerase chain reaction technique. Cancer Res. 1991;51:3497–502.

Index

Falk Symposium Series

43. Reutter W, Popper H, Arias IM, Heinrich PC, Keppler D, Landmann L, eds.: *Modulation of Liver Cell Expression*. Falk Symposium No. 43. 1987 ISBN: 0-85200-677-2*
44. Boyer JL, Bianchi L, eds.: *Liver Cirrhosis*. Falk Symposium No. 44. 1987 ISBN: 0-85200-993-3*
45. Paumgartner G, Stiehl A, Gerok W, eds.: *Bile Acids and the Liver*. Falk Symposium No. 45. 1987 ISBN: 0-85200-675-6*
46. Goebell H, Peskar BM, Malchow H, eds.: *Inflammatory Bowel Diseases – Basic Research & Clinical Implications*. Falk Symposium No. 46. 1988 ISBN: 0-7462-0067-6*
47. Bianchi L, Holt P, James OFW, Butler RN, eds.: *Aging in Liver and Gastrointestinal Tract*. Falk Symposium No. 47. 1988 ISBN: 0-7462-0066-8*
48. Heilmann C, ed.: *Calcium-Dependent Processes in the Liver*. Falk Symposium No. 48. 1988 ISBN: 0-7462-0075-7*
50. Singer MV, Goebell H, eds.: *Nerves and the Gastrointestinal Tract*. Falk Symposium No. 50. 1989 ISBN: 0-7462-0114-1
51. Bannasch P, Keppler D, Weber G, eds.: *Liver Cell Carcinoma*. Falk Symposium No. 51. 1989 ISBN: 0-7462-0111-7
52. Paumgartner G, Stiehl A, Gerok W, eds.: *Trends in Bile Acid Research*. Falk Symposium No. 52. 1989 ISBN: 0-7462-0112-5
53. Paumgartner G, Stiehl A, Barbara L, Roda E, eds.: *Strategies for the Treatment of Hepatobiliary Diseases*. Falk Symposium No. 53. 1990 ISBN: 0-7923-8903-4
54. Bianchi L, Gerok W, Maier K-P, Deinhardt F, eds.: *Infectious Diseases of the Liver*. Falk Symposium No. 54. 1990 ISBN: 0-7923-8902-6
55. Falk Symposium No. 55 not published

55B. Hadziselimovic F, Herzog B, Bürgin-Wolff A, eds.: *Inflammatory Bowel Disease and Coeliac Disease in Children*. International Falk Symposium. 1990 ISBN 0-7462-0125-7

56. Williams CN, eds.: *Trends in Inflammatory Bowel Disease Therapy*. Falk Symposium No. 56. 1990 ISBN: 0-7923-8952-2
57. Bock KW, Gerok W, Matern S, Schmid R, eds.: *Hepatic Metabolism and Disposition of Endo- and Xenobiotics*. Falk Symposium No. 57. 1991 ISBN: 0-7923-8953-0
58. Paumgartner G, Stiehl A, Gerok W, eds.: *Bile Acids as Therapeutic Agents: From Basic Science to Clinical Practice*. Falk Symposium No. 58. 1991 ISBN: 0-7923-8954-9
59. Halter F, Garner A, Tytgat GNJ, eds.: *Mechanisms of Peptic Ulcer Healing*. Falk Symposium No. 59. 1991 ISBN: 0-7923-8955-7
60. Goebell H, Ewe K, Malchow H, Koelbel Ch, eds.: *Inflammatory Bowel Diseases – Progress in Basic Research and Clinical Implications*. Falk Symposium No. 60. 1991 ISBN: 0-7923-8956-5
61. Falk Symposium No. 61 not published
62. Dowling RH, Folsch UR, Löser Ch, eds.: *Polyamines in the Gastrointestinal Tract*. Falk Symposium No. 62. 1992 ISBN: 0-7923-8976-X
63. Lentze MJ, Reichen J, eds.: *Paediatric Cholestasis: Novel Approaches to Treatment*. Falk Symposium No. 63. 1992 ISBN: 0-7923-8977-8
64. Demling L, Frühmorgen P, eds.: *Non-Neoplastic Diseases of the Anorectum*. Falk Symposium No. 64. 1992 ISBN: 0-7923-8979-4

64B. Gressner AM, Ramadori G, eds.: *Molecular and Cell Biology of Liver Fibrogenesis*. International Falk Symposium. 1992 ISBN: 0-7923-8980-8

*These titles were published under the MTP Press imprint.

65. Hadziselimovic F, Herzog B, eds.: *Inflammatory Bowel Diseases and Morbus Hirschprung*. Falk Symposium No. 65. 1992 ISBN: 0-7923-8995-6
66. Martin F, McLeod RS, Sutherland LR, Williams CN, eds.: *Trends in Inflammatory Bowel Disease Therapy*. Falk Symposium No. 66. 1993 ISBN: 0-7923-8827-5
67. Schölmerich J, Kruis W, Goebell H, Hohenberger W, Gross V, eds.: *Inflammatory Bowel Diseases – Pathophysiology as Basis of Treatment*. Falk Symposium No. 67. 1993 ISBN: 0-7923-8996-4
68. Paumgartner G, Stiehl A, Gerok W, eds.: *Bile Acids and The Hepatobiliary System: From Basic Science to Clinical Practice*. Falk Symposium No. 68. 1993 ISBN: 0-7923-8829-1
69. Schmid R, Bianchi L, Gerok W, Maier K-P, eds.: *Extrahepatic Manifestations in Liver Diseases*. Falk Symposium No. 69. 1993 ISBN: 0-7923-8821-6
70. Meyer zum Büschenfelde K-H, Hoofnagle J, Manns M, eds.: *Immunology and Liver*. Falk Symposium No. 70. 1993 ISBN: 0-7923-8830-5
71. Surrenti C, Casini A, Milani S, Pinzani M , eds.: *Fat-Storing Cells and Liver Fibrosis*. Falk Symposium No. 71. 1994 ISBN: 0-7923-8842-9
72. Rachmilewitz D, ed.: *Inflammatory Bowel Diseases – 1994*. Falk Symposium No. 72. 1994 ISBN: 0-7923-8845-3
73. Binder HJ, Cummings J, Soergel KH, eds.: *Short Chain Fatty Acids*. Falk Symposium No. 73. 1994 ISBN: 0-7923-8849-6

73B. Möllmann HW, May B, eds.: *Glucocorticoid Therapy in Chronic Inflammatory Bowel Disease: from basic principles to rational therapy*. International Falk Workshop. 1996 ISBN 0-7923-8708-2

74. Keppler D, Jungermann K, eds.: *Transport in the Liver*. Falk Symposium No. 74. 1994 ISBN: 0-7923-8858-5

74B. Stange EF, ed.: *Chronic Inflammatory Bowel Disease*. Falk Symposium. 1995 ISBN: 0-7923-8876-3

75. van Berge Henegouwen GP, van Hoek B, De Groote J, Matern S, Stockbrügger RW, eds.: *Cholestatic Liver Diseases: New Strategies for Prevention and Treatment of Hepatobiliary and Cholestatic Liver Diseases*. Falk Symposium 75. 1994. ISBN: 0-7923-8867-4
76. Monteiro E, Tavarela Veloso F, eds.: *Inflammatory Bowel Diseases: New Insights into Mechanisms of Inflammation and Challenges in Diagnosis and Treatment*. Falk Symposium 76. 1995. ISBN 0-7923-8884-4
77. Singer MV, Ziegler R, Rohr G, eds.: *Gastrointestinal Tract and Endocrine System*. Falk Symposium 77. 1995. ISBN 0-7923-8877-1
78. Decker K, Gerok W, Andus T, Gross V, eds.: *Cytokines and the Liver*. Falk Symposium 78. 1995. ISBN 0-7923-8878-X
79. Holstege A, Schölmerich J, Hahn EG, eds.: *Portal Hypertension*. Falk Symposium 79. 1995. ISBN 0-7923-8879-8
80. Hofmann AF, Paumgartner G, Stiehl A, eds.: *Bile Acids in Gastroenterology: Basic and Clinical Aspects*. Falk Symposium 80. 1995 ISBN 0-7923-8880-1
81. Riecken EO, Stallmach A, Zeitz M, Heise W, eds.: *Malignancy and Chronic Inflammation in the Gastrointestinal Tract – New Concepts*. Falk Symposium 81. 1995 ISBN 0-7923-8889-5
82. Fleig WE, ed.: *Inflammatory Bowel Diseases: New Developments and Standards*. Falk Symposium 82. 1995 ISBN 0-7923-8890-6

Falk Symposium Series

82B. Paumgartner G, Beuers U, eds.: *Bile Acids in Liver Diseases.* International Falk Workshop. 1995 ISBN 0-7923-8891-7

83. Dobrilla G, Felder M, de Pretis G, eds.: *Advances in Hepatobiliary and Pancreatic Diseases: Special Clinical Topics.* Falk Symposium 83. 1995. ISBN 0-7923-8892-5

84. Fromm H, Leuschner U, eds.: *Bile Acids – Cholestasis – Gallstones: Advances in Basic and Clinical Bile Acid Research.* Falk Symposium 84. 1995 ISBN 0-7923-8893-3

85. Tytgat GNJ, Bartelsman JFWM, van Deventer SJH, eds.: *Inflammatory Bowel Diseases.* Falk Symposium 85. 1995 ISBN 0-7923-8894-1

86. Berg PA, Leuschner U, eds.: *Bile Acids and Immunology.* Falk Symposium 86. 1996 ISBN 0-7923-8700-7

87. Schmid R, Bianchi L, Blum HE, Gerok W, Maier KP, Stalder GA, eds.: *Acute and Chronic Liver Diseases: Molecular Biology and Clinics.* Falk Symposium 87. 1996 ISBN 0-7923-8701-5

88. Blum HE, Wu GY, Wu CH, eds.: *Molecular Diagnosis and Gene Therapy.* Falk Symposium 88. 1996 ISBN 0-7923-8702-3

88B. Poupon RE, Reichen J, eds.: *Surrogate Markers to Assess Efficacy of TReatment in Chronic Liver Diseases.* International Falk Workshop. 1996 ISBN 0-7923-8705-8

89. Reyes HB, Leuschner U, Arias IM, eds.: *Pregnancy, Sex Hormones and the Liver.* Falk Symposium 89. 1996 ISBN 0-7923-8704-X

89B. Broelsch CE, Burdelski M, Rogiers X, eds.: *Cholestatic Liver Diseases in Children and Adults.* International Falk Workshop. 1996 ISBN 0-7923-8710-4

90. Lam S-K, Paumgartner P, Wang B, eds.: *Update on Hepatobiliary Diseases 1996.* Falk Symposium 90. 1996 ISBN 0-7923-8715-5

91. Hadziselimovic F, Herzog B, eds.: *Inflammatory Bowel Diseases and Chronic Recurrent Abdominal Pain.* Falk Symposium 91. 1996 ISBN 0-7923-8722-8

91B. Alvaro D, Benedetti A, Strazzabosco M, eds.: *Vanishing Bile Duct Syndrome – Pathophysiology and Treatment.* International Falk Workshop. 1996 ISBN 0-7923-8721-X

92. Gerok W, Loginov AS, Pokrowskij VI, eds.: *New Trends in Hepatology 1996.* Falk Symposium 92. 1997 ISBN 0-7923-8723-6

93. Paumgartner G, Stiehl A, Gerok W, eds.: *Bile Acids in Hepatobiliary Diseases – Basic Research and Clinical Application.* Falk Symposium 93. 1997 ISBN 0-7923-8725-2

94. Halter F, Winton D, Wright NA, eds.: *The Gut as a Model in Cell and Molecular Biology.* Falk Symposium 94. 1997 ISBN 0-7923-8726-0

94B. Kruse-Jarres JD, Schölmerich J, eds.: *Zinc and Diseases of the Digestive Tract.* International Falk Workshop. 1997 ISBN 0-7923-8724-4

95. Ewe K, Eckardt VF, Enck P, eds.: *Constipation and Anorectal Insufficiency.* Falk Symposium 95. 1997 ISBN 0-7923-8727-9

96. Andus T, Goebell H, Layer P, Schölmerich J, eds.: *Inflammatory Bowel Disease – from Bench to Bedside.* Falk Symposium 96. 1997 ISBN 0-7923-8728-7

97. Campieri M, Bianchi-Porro G, Fiocchi C, Schölmerich J, eds. *Clinical Challenges in Inflammatory Bowel Diseases: Diagnosis, Prognosis and Treatment.* Falk Symposium 97. 1998 ISBN 0-7923-8733-3

98. Lembcke B, Kruis W, Sartor RB, eds. *Systemic Manifestations of IBD: The Pending Challenge for Subtle Diagnosis and Treatment.* Falk Symposium 98. 1998 ISBN 0-7923-8734-1

Falk Symposium Series

99. Goebell H, Holtmann G, Talley NJ, eds. *Functional Dyspepsia and Irritable Bowel Syndrome: Concepts and Controversies.* Falk Symposium 99. 1998 ISBN 0-7923-8735-X
100. Blum HE, Bode Ch, Bode JCh, Sartor RB, eds. *Gut and the Liver.* Falk Symposium 100. 1998 ISBN 0-7923-8736-8
101. Rachmilewitz D, ed. *V International Symposium on Inflammatory Bowel Diseases.* Falk Symposium 101. 1998 ISBN 0-7923-8743-0
102. Manns MP, Boyer JL, Jansen PLM, Reichen J, eds. *Cholestatic Liver Diseases.* Falk Symposium 102. 1998 ISBN 0-7923-8746-5

102B. Manns MP, Chapman RW, Stiehl A, Wiesner R, eds. *Primary Sclerosing Cholangitis.* International Falk Workshop. 1998. ISBN 0-7923-8745-7

103. Häussinger D, Jungermann K, eds. *Liver and Nervous System.* Falk Symposium 102. 1998 ISBN 0-7924-8742-2

103B. Häussinger D, Heinrich PC, eds. *Signalling in the Liver.* International Falk Workshop. 1998 ISBN 0-7923-8744-9

www.ingramcontent.com/pod-product-compliance
Ingram Content Group UK Ltd.
Pitfield, Milton Keynes, MK11 3LW, UK
UKHW020137160926
475607UK00003B/88
* 9 7 8 0 7 9 2 3 8 7 4 5 9 *